ACCELERATED ORTHODONTICS

MODERN TECHNIQUES & INNOVATIONS FOR FASTER TOOTH MOVEMENT

DR. ARUN V R
DR. DEEPAK C
DR. DEENADAYALAN P
DR. AKSHAY TANDON
DR. NIDHI ANGRISH

Made with ♥ on the Notion Press Platform
www.notionpress.com

To my parents, who gave me the roots to grow and the courage to dream.

Every word on these pages exists because you believed in me first.

Contents

Acknowledgements

I take this opportunity to express my profound sense of gratitude to all those who have supported, guided, and inspired me throughout the completion of my library dissertation. This academic endeavour has been a journey of learning, reflection, and growth, and its successful completion stands as a testament to the collective encouragement and guidance I have received from many individuals.

Foremost, I express my sincere and heartfelt gratitude to my esteemed guide, **Prof. Dr. C. Deepak,** MDS, FDS (RCPS Glasgow), DIBO, PhD, Head of the Department of Orthodontics and Dentofacial Orthopaedics, S.R.M. Kattankulathur Dental College and Hospital (SRMKDC), SRM Institute of Science and Technology. His exemplary leadership, profound knowledge, and unwavering support have been instrumental in shaping this dissertation. His insightful guidance, constructive criticism, and constant motivation provided a strong academic foundation and encouraged me to strive for intellectual excellence.

I am deeply indebted to **Dr. Deenadayalan P,** MDS, Professor, Department of Orthodontics and Dentofacial Orthopaedics, SRMKDC, for his patience, encouragement, and valuable mentorship throughout this challenging yet rewarding journey. His guidance has been a source of confidence and clarity at every stage of this work.

I am grateful to **Dr. Akshay Tandon,** MDS, AssociateProfessor, Department of Orthodontics and Dentofacial Orthopaedics, SRMKDC, for his insightful suggestions, scholarly mentorship, and constant encouragement, which greatly enhanced my understanding of the subject.

I extend my sincere gratitude to the esteemed faculty members of the Department of Orthodontics and Dentofacial Orthopaedics, SRMKDC. I express my appreciation to **Dr. Nidhi Angrish** (Assistant Professor) for her keen attention to detail and thoughtful feedback, which significantly improved the academic quality of this dissertation. I also thank **Dr. K. Praveen** (Assistant Professor) for his dedication, professional guidance, and consistent support, which contributed immensely to my academic development. I am equally thankful to **Dr. Reshma Mohan** (Assistant Professor) for her encouragement and guidance, which helped broaden my perspectives and strengthen my approach to the subject.

I extend my sincere appreciation to the non-teaching staff of the department and the library staff for their indispensable assistance. Their efforts in facilitating access to academic resources, managing administrative responsibilities, and providing technical support ensured a smooth and efficient research process.

I also express my gratitude to my peers **Dr. Hariis M** and **Dr. Nayana Setty** my seniors **Dr. Reshma Kishor Kumar, Dr. Sanjivani Shukla, Dr. Bharathi Priya** and **Dr. Manjula**and my juniors **Dr. Varun, Dr. Adarsh** and **Dr. Pavithra** for their camaraderie, encouragement, and collaborative spirit. The exchange of ideas, discussions, and shared learning experiences with them made this academic journey enriching and memorable.

Above all, I extend my deepest gratitude to my family. I am immensely thankful to my parents, **Mr. Rajan V B** and **Mrs. Nisha G**, for their unconditional love, patience, and unwavering support, which strengthened my resolve during the most demanding phases of this journey.

Above all, I bow in reverence to **Almighty Lord Shiva**, whose divine blessings, inner strength, and guidance enabled me to persevere through challenges and accomplish this academic milestone.

This dissertation is not merely a reflection of my individual effort but a culmination of the guidance, encouragement, and support bestowed upon me by all those mentioned above. I remain deeply grateful to each one of them.

Dr. ARUN V R
Postgraduate
Department of Orthodontics and Dentofacial Orthopaedics
SRM Kattankulathur Dental College and Hospital
SRM Institute of Science and Technology

Prologue

For many years, orthodontics has been constrained by a significant anatomical limitation: the rigid confines of the alveolar housing. Despite our advancements in bracket designs, archwire materials, and intricate biomechanics, we have always been wary of the cortical plates. The risks of fenestrations, dehiscences, and periodontal issues have set our boundaries, with time being our sole means to contend with the dense cortical bone.

However, bone is not an immovable barrier; it is a dynamic tissue that can be surgically modified. The transition from purely mechanical orthodontics to Surgically Facilitated Orthodontic Therapy (SFOT) represents a major clinical advancement in our field. We are no longer just applying forces to teeth and waiting for the periodontium to gradually adapt. Now, we are directly intervening at the surgical level to alter the alveolar matrix itself.

By intentionally utilizing the Regional Acceleratory Phenomenon (RAP) through specific alveolar decortication and corticotomies, we create a temporary state of osteopenia. This localized biological trauma significantly lowers tissue resistance, enabling rapid and efficient tooth movement. Moreover, when these surgical interventions are paired with particulate bone grafting—as seen in Periodontally Accelerated Osteogenic Orthodontics (PAOO)—we achieve something historically unique: we not only move teeth faster but also enhance the periodontium. We enlarge the anatomical space, thicken the biotype, and improve the long-term stability of the final occlusion.

This book is devoted to the powerful convergence of oral surgery, periodontics, and advanced orthodontic biomechanics. It is crafted to be a thorough, evidence-based resource on the surgical protocols that free clinicians from traditional biological limitations. In the following chapters, we will connect the dots between surgical tools and orthodontic wires, outlining the techniques needed to perform everything from localized micro-osteoperforations to full-arch decortication and grafting.

The quest for clinical excellence requires us to look beyond the bracket slot. By mastering the surgical alteration of the alveolar housing, we provide our patients with more than just significantly reduced treatment times—we offer them safer biomechanics, expanded correction possibilities, and improved periodontal health. The future of orthodontics is inherently interdisciplinary. Welcome to the surgical frontier.

CHAPTER I

INTRODUCTION

Before beginning orthodontic treatment, patients are primarily concernedwith the duration of the process. Over the last two decades, advancements in devices and methods have made orthodontics more efficient, though not necessarily quicker. Numerous innovations have been made to enhance bracket design and treatment protocols; however, the only proven methods to accelerate tooth movement through the alveolar bone require significant surgical procedures. As with any medical treatment, prolonged duration increases the risk of side effects and unsatisfactory results. By reducing the length of treatment, patients can avoid the common complications associated with long-term orthodontic care. The risk of decalcification, which can result in "white lesions" due to prolonged banding, is minimized. Additionally, root blunting is lessened with shorter treatment periods. A reduced treatment time allows patients to resume their regular oral hygiene practices and keep their teeth clean[1].

Traditional orthodontic treatment has typically been linked to lengthy durations, often spanning from 18 to 36 months[2]. In the past, the duration of treatment was largely determined by biological factors such as the rate of bone turnover, the response of the periodontal ligament (PDL), and the natural limits of tooth movement. Early orthodontic innovators, like Edward H. Angle focused on mechanical accuracy but regarded the slow biological responses as inevitable.

Accelerated orthodontics encompasses a range of clinical techniques, technologies, and biological strategies designed to decrease the overall duration of treatment while maintaining the quality of outcomes, stability, and periodontal health. The primary rationale is to enhance the rate of bone remodeling, specifically osteoclastic and osteoblastic activity, surrounding the moving tooth[3].

To date, several innovative approaches have been documented to expedite orthodontic tooth movement, including low-level laser therapy, pulsed electromagnetic fields, electrical currents, corticotomy, distraction osteogenesis, and mechanical vibration[4].

Orthodontic tooth movement involves the physiological adaptation of alveolar bone to mechanical strains, accompanied by minor reversible injury to the periodontium. Under normal, healthy conditions, this movement is facilitated by highly coordinated and efficient bone remodeling, necessitating the coupling of bone formation with bone resorption. The classical pressure-tension theory posits that chemical signals, rather than electrical ones, serve as the stimulus for cellular differentiation and, ultimately, tooth movement. According to this theory, within seconds of force application, the tooth shifts its position within the periodontal ligament (PDL) space, resulting in PDL compression in certain areas and PDL stretch or tension in others. While blood flow decreases on the compression side, it is maintained or increased on the tension side. If the force is sustained, the alteration in blood flow rapidly (within minutes) changes the oxygen tension (O_2:CO_2 level) and the chemical environment by releasing biologically active agents such as prostaglandins and cytokines (e.g., Interleukin (IL)-1b). These chemical mediators differentially influence cellular activities in the compression versus tension areas within the PDL, promoting a net outcome of bone resorption on the compression side and bone formation on the tension side. The magnitude of force is associated with varied cellular responses on the compression side. Heavy force interrupts blood flow, leading to cell death under compression (hyalinization). Consequently, no osteoclast differentiation occurs within the compressed PDL space; instead, a delayed recruitment and differentiation of osteoclasts from adjacent bone marrow space is responsible for the "undermining resorption" that removes the lamina dura adjacent to the compressed PDL. Tooth movement ensues following the completion of these processes on the compression side, but not before. Therefore, it typically takes 7 to 14 days for tooth movement to occur when heavy force is applied. In contrast, light force only reduces blood flow, allowing for the rapid recruitment of osteoclasts either locally within the PDL or via blood flow. These osteoclasts remove the lamina dura through the process of "frontal resorption"[5].

Tooth movement typically starts shortly after, generally within two days following the application of light force. Clinically, it is nearly impossible to completely prevent blood vessel occlusion, so some degree of hyalinization always occurs, resulting in tooth movement through a combination of undermining and frontal resorption. As previously mentioned, orthodontic loading affects blood flow in the periodontal ligament (PDL), leading to regional hypoxia. The decrease in oxygen tension stabilizes hypoxia-inducible factor-1 (HIF-1), a transcription factor that activates the expression of vascular endothelial growth factor (VEGF) and RANKL in PDL fibroblasts and osteoblasts, which also increases osteoclast differentiation, promoting resorption in compressed areas. Under mild hypoxia, HIF-1 encourages cell proliferation and angiogenesis downstream of VEGF, aiding in the regeneration of the PDL and its blood supply. Hypoxia is a crucial trigger for orthodontic tissue remodeling, working alongside loading-induced fluid flow, another signaling activator. The fluid flow hypothesis emphasizes the response of osteocytes and fibroblasts to strain caused by fluid movement in canaliculi.

The application of force initiates a series of events, including: 1) matrix strain and fluid flow; 2) cell strain; 3) cell activation and differentiation; and 4) tissue remodeling. Mechanoreceptor cells that detect strain are found in the bone as osteocytes and in the PDL as fibroblasts. Loading leads to the remodeling of mineralized tissue (bone) and non-mineralized paradental tissues (the PDL, gingiva, and neurovascular supply). When teeth are loaded, interstitial fluid is pushed through the canaliculi and around osteocytes, causing strain on the cell surface and extracellular matrix. The extracellular matrix (ECM) of bone is a hydroxyapatite-collagen composite, while the ECM of the PDL is a network of fibrous structural proteins embedded in a polysaccharide gel surrounding cells. Fluid flow applies shear stress to the bone ECM and cell membrane, disrupting integrins and activating signaling cascades in osteocytes. Integrins are transmembrane proteins that connect a cell's external ECM to its internal cytoskeleton. Stimulation of integrins on the cell surface leads to the release of intracellular molecules that change osteocyte gene expression, promoting the differentiation of osteoblasts and osteoclasts to form and resorb bone. Intracellular calcium levels rise, increasing phospholipase A activity, which releases arachidonic acid, the precursor to prostaglandins; cyclooxygenase (COX) enzymes then convert arachidonic acid to prostaglandins, key inflammatory mediators. Second messengers cAMP and cGMP are elevated downstream of calcium, triggering phosphorylation events and subsequent changes in gene expression with the release of autocrine and paracrine signals initiating bone turnover. Osteocytes are mechanosensors that link strain from orthodontic loading to tissue remodeling. Fibroblasts perform a similar mechanosensor function in the PDL and gingiva. Strain disrupts the ECM in the PDL and gingiva. Like osteocytes, fibroblasts express transmembrane integrin receptors. Stress from mechanical loading is transmitted intracellularly from the ECM via integrins, which induce a signaling cascade through focal adhesion kinases (FAK) to alter gene expression, cytoskeletal organization, proliferation, and differentiation, ultimately leading to tissue remodeling [5].

Accelerated orthodontics signifies a transformative approach that amalgamates biological principles, technological advancements, and biomechanical strategies to facilitate expedited and more effective tooth movement. As patient expectations continue to evolve, it is imperative for clinicians to remain well-versed in evidence-based methodologies, including their indications and limitations. This introduction offers essential knowledge, laying the groundwork for a comprehensive examination of the scientific principles, techniques, clinical protocols, and prospective innovations that characterize accelerated orthodontics.

CHAPTER II

REVIEW OF LITERATURE

Köle H[6] in 1959 done seminal work on the evolution of corticotomy-facilitated orthodontics was published, positing that the continuity and thickness of the denser cortical bone layer presented the greatest resistance to tooth movement. He hypothesized that by disrupting the continuity of this cortical layer, he was effectively creating and mobilizing blocks of bone in which teeth were embedded, a concept he termed bony block movement. Kole reported that significant active tooth movements were achieved within 6 to 12 weeks. He employed vertical wedge-shaped crestal ostectomies, leaving only a thin layer of bone over the proximal root surfaces of adjacent teeth. Furthermore, he noted that after 6 to 8 months of retention, the corticotomy-facilitated orthodontic cases exhibited remarkable stability.

Herald Frost[7] in 1983 identified that surgical trauma to osseous tissue induces significant reorganization activity in the vicinity of the injury site, particularly in osseous and soft tissue surgery. He collectively termed this sequence of physiological healing events as the "Regional Acceleratory Phenomenon" (RAP). RAP represents a localized tissue response to harmful stimuli, facilitating accelerated tissue regeneration within a regional regeneration and remodeling process. The duration, extent, and intensity of this response are directly proportional to the magnitude of the stimulus. The duration of RAP is contingent upon the type of tissue involved and typically persists for approximately four months in human bone. This phenomenon results in bone healing occurring at a rate 10 to 50 times faster than normal bone turnover. The healing phases of RAP have been investigated in the rat tibia. A cortical bridge of woven bone, a fundamental component of RAP, provides mechanical stability to the bone post-injury. From the seventh day, the woven bone in the cortical area begins remodeling into lamellar bone, while the woven bone in the medullary area undergoes resorption, leading to temporary local osteopenia. It appears that medullary bone requires reorganization and reconstruction following the establishment of the new cortical bone structure and must adapt to the reestablishment of cortical integrity, which occurs over three weeks in rats. Additionally, there exists a Systemic Acceleratory Phenomenon (SAP) of osteogenesis, attributed to the systemic release of humoral factors.

Yamasaki et al.[8] in 1984 conducted a study in which they administered chemically synthesized prostaglandin E1 (PGEI) in clinical cases involving orthodontic tooth movement. The findings indicated that the rate of distal canine movement was approximately 1.6 times greater on the side receiving PGEI injections compared to the side injected with a vehicle. Throughout the study, no macroscopic side effects were observed in the gingiva, nor were any roentgenographic changes detected in the alveolar bone, aside from a slight pain reaction consistent with orthodontic tooth movement.

Anholm et al.[9] in 1986 posited that following the demineralization of the alveolar housing over the root surfaces, a soft tissue matrix of the bone, which could accompany the root and subsequently undergo remineralization, emerges upon the completion of orthodontic treatment. To augment bony volumes subsequent to the application of orthodontic forces, they advocated for the utilization of particulate bone grafting in conjunction with decortication procedures.

Gantes B et al.[10] in 1990 detailed the corticotomy surgical technique employed in conjunction with orthodontic therapy, examining its impact on the periodontal status of the affected teeth. The surgical procedure involved intracrevicular incisions and the elevation of buccal and lingual mucoperiosteal flaps. Subsequently, buccal and lingual vertical grooves were created, penetrating the cortical bone between the roots. These grooves extended from just below the interproximal alveolar bone margin to beyond the apical levels of the teeth. Buccal and lingual horizontal grooves connected the apical extensions of the vertical grooves. The orthodontic appliance was activated immediately following wound closure. Plaque scores, probing depths, and probing attachment levels were recorded prior to the surgical procedure and after the completion of orthodontic treatment in five patients. The findings indicated that the corticotomy procedure resulted in minimal changes to the periodontal attachment apparatus.

M Saito et al.[11] in 1991 investigated the role of cytokines as local mediators released by immune system cells in response to various stimuli. These polypeptides may interact with bone cells either directly or indirectly. The findings indicate that periodontal ligament cells exhibit an increased production of PGE in response to mechanical stress, and that this response is further enhanced by IL-1 beta.

W S Simonet et al.[12] in 1997 introduced a glycoprotein that plays a regulatory role in bone resorption. This protein, identified as Osteoprotegerin (OPG), is a novel member of the tumor necrosis factor

(TNF) receptor superfamily. The findings indicate that OPG functions as a soluble factor in the regulation of bone mass, suggesting its potential application in the treatment of osteoporosis associated with increased osteoclast activity.

E J Liou et al.[13] in 1998 investigated the process of osteogenesis within the periodontal ligament during orthodontic tooth movement, finding it analogous to osteogenesis in the midpalatal suture during rapid palatal expansion. They introduced the concept of "distracting the periodontal ligament" to achieve rapid canine retraction within three weeks, termed dental distraction. During this process, 73% of the first molars did not exhibit mesial movement, while 27% moved less than 0.5 mm mesially within the same period. Radiographic examination indicated minimal apical or lateral surface root resorption of the canine. The authors concluded that the periodontal ligament could be rapidly distracted without complications.

M K Collins et al.[14] in 1998 conducted a study to ascertain whether the rate and extent of orthodontic tooth movement in a sample of cats could be augmented through the injection of the vitamin D metabolite 1,25-dihydroxycholecalciferol (1,25D) into the periodontal ligament. Following a 21-day period of canine retraction using a light-wire retraction spring, the teeth that received weekly intraligamentous injections of a 1,25D solution in dimethylsulfoxide (DMSO) exhibited a 60% greater movement compared to matched control teeth (P < 0.05). Histological analysis revealed an increased recruitment and activation of mononuclear osteoclasts, leading to enhanced alveolar bone resorption on the pressure side of the periodontal ligament. No discernible clinical, microscopic, or biochemical side effects were observed.

S Soma et al.[15] in 2000 conducted a study to determine whether the local and chronic administration of PTH(1-34) could expedite orthodontic tooth movement. The findings indicated that the local injection of PTH in a slow-release formulation is applicable to orthodontic therapy.

W M Wilcko et al.[16] in 2001 showed two case reports demonstrating a new orthodontic method offering short treatment times and ability to reshape and increase buccolingual thickness of supporting alveolar bone. A 24-year-old man with Class I severely crowded malocclusion and constricted maxilla with posterior crossbites and a 17-year-old female with Class I moderately to severely crowded malocclusion requested shortened orthodontic treatment times. The surgery technique included buccal and lingual full-thickness flaps, selective partial decortication of cortical plates, bone grafting/augmentation, and primary flap closure. Following surgery, orthodontic adjustments were made every 2 weeks. Both cases were completed in approximately 6 months and 2 weeks. Posttreatment evaluation revealed good results. At 15 months following surgery in one patient, a full-thickness flap was reflected. Visual examination showed good maintenance of alveolar crest height and increased buccal bone thickness. The canine and premolars were expanded buccally by more than 3 mm, with an increase in buccolingual thickness of overlying buccal bone. A preexisting bony fenestration buccal of the first premolar root was covered. These findings support incorporating bone augmentation into corticotomy surgery, enabling completion of orthodontic treatment with a more intact periodontium. The rapid expansive tooth movements without significant apical root resorption may be attributed to the osteoclastic phase of the regional acceleratory phenomenon. Instead of bony "block" movement or resorption/apposition, the degree of demineralization/remineralization might better explain what occurs in alveolar bone during physiologic tooth movement in these patients.

Takahiro Oshiro et al.[17] in 2002 proposed that osteoprotegerin (OPG) and receptor activator of nuclear factor kappa-B ligand (RANKL) play a role in the remodeling of alveolar bone during orthodontic tooth movement. Their study found no significant difference in the intensity of RANKL expression between OPG (+/+) littermates and OPG-deficient mice. In both wild-type and OPG-deficient mice, RANKL protein expression was observed in osteoblasts, fibroblasts, and osteoclasts, predominantly located in resorption lacunae. These findings indicate that during orthodontic tooth movement, RANKL and OPG within periodontal tissues are crucial determinants in regulating balanced alveolar bone resorption.

Ali Reza Sekhavat et al.[18] in 2002 studied the effects of oral misoprostol on orthodontic tooth movement and root resorption in rats. Results showed oral misoprostol increased orthodontic tooth movement in experimental groups compared to controls, with statistical significance at doses of 10.0-100.0 microg/kg (P <.001). No significant differences existed among these doses or in root resorption between groups, though root resorption showed an increasing trend. These findings suggest oral misoprostol can enhance orthodontic tooth movement with minimal root resorption.

Massoud Seifi et al.[19] in 2003 conducted a study to assess potential alterations in orthodontic tooth movement (OTM) and root resorption resulting from local injections of prostaglandin E2 (PGE2), both independently and in conjunction with calcium gluconate (Ca). The findings underscore the critical role of calcium ions in conjunction with PGE2 in mitigating root resorption while markedly enhancing orthodontic tooth movement.

Selin Kale et al.[20] in 2004 conducted a study to compare the effects of local administrations of prostaglandin E2 (PGE2) and 1,25-dihydroxycholecalciferol (1,25-DHCC) on orthodontic tooth movement in rats. Both PGE2 and 1,25-DHCC were found to increase the extent of tooth movement over a 9-day experimental period without any detectable adverse effects. This increase is considered clinically significant.

Seher Sayin et al.[21] in 2004 said rapid canine distalization through periodontal ligament distraction resembles midpalatal suture distraction during rapid palatal expansion, achievable in three weeks. This study evaluated effects of rapid canine distalization on dentoalveolar tissues using semirigid tooth-borne distractors. The study included 43 canine teeth in 18 patients requiring first premolar extractions, with a mean age of 16.7 years. Second premolars and first molars served as anchors. Orthodontic records were taken before treatment and after consolidation. Periapical radiographs were obtained weekly during distalization. Distractors were activated 0.25 mm thrice daily, completing distalization in three weeks. Within-group differences were evaluated using the Wilcoxon test. Maxillary canines were distalized 5.76 mm with 11.47 degrees distal tipping, while first molars moved mesially 0.56 mm and extruded 0.64 mm. Maxillary incisors showed 1.44 degrees palatal tipping. Mandibular canines moved distally 3.5 mm with 7.16 degrees tipping, with no anchorage loss in mandibular first molars.

Delma R Cruz et al.[22] in 2004 conducted 11 patients participating in a 2-month study of low intensity laser therapy (LILT). One half of the upper arcade served as control group (CG) with mechanical activation of canine teeth every 30 days. The opposite half received mechanical activation and diode laser irradiation at 780 nm, for 10 seconds at 20 mW, 5 J/cm2, on 4 days monthly. Biometrical progress data were statistically compared. Results showed significantly higher acceleration of canine retraction on the LILT-treated side versus control. The findings indicated LILT accelerates teeth movement and could shorten treatment duration.

Haluk Işeri et al.[23] in 2005 introduced an innovative technique for rapid canine retraction utilizing distraction osteogenesis. This article presents the effects of dentoalveolar distraction on dentofacial structures. Complete retraction of the canines was achieved in an average duration of 10.05 (+/-2.01) days. The authors concluded that the dentoalveolar distraction technique is a novel method that significantly reduces the overall orthodontic treatment time by approximately 50% without adverse effects on the surrounding structures.

Y Nishijima et al.[24] in 2006 conducted a study to ascertain the levels of receptor activator of NFkB ligand (RANKL) and osteoprotegerin (OPG) in gingival crevicular fluid (GCF) during orthodontic tooth movement. A secondary objective was to examine the impact of compression force on the production of RANKL and OPG by human periodontal ligament (hPDL) cells. The findings suggest that variations in the levels of RANKL and OPG may play a role in bone resorption as a response to compression force.

Carlos Sechi Goulart et al.[25] in 2006 conducted a double-blind study to evaluate the effect of gallium-aluminum-arsenic (GaAlAs) laser irradiation on the rate of orthodontic movement in canine premolars.The findings suggest that photoradiation may accelerate orthodontic movement at a dosage of 5.25 J/cm^2,whereas a higher dosage of 35.0 J/cm^2 may impede it.

W Limpanichkul et al.[26] in 2006 investigated the hypothesis that the combination of mechanical forces and low-level laser therapy could enhance the rate of orthodontic tooth movement. Their findings indicated that the energy density of low-level laser therapy applied at the surface level in this study (25 J/cm^2) was likely insufficient to produce either a stimulatory or inhibitory effect on the rate of orthodontic tooth movement.

H Kanzaki et al.[27] in 2006 reported that selective alveolar-bone resorption and receptor activator of nuclear factor kappa B ligand (RANKL) expression is induced on the compressed side of an orthodontically moving tooth. They found that every-3-days OPG gene transfer to periodontal-tissue inhibited RANKL-mediated osteoclastogenesis and reduced experimental tooth movement. They showed that RANKL gene transfer to periodontal-tissue activated osteoclastogenesis and accelerated experimental tooth movement. Local RANKL gene transfer might be useful for shortening orthodontic treatment and moving ankylosed teeth where teeth fuse to surrounding bone.

Vinod Krishnan et al.[28] in 2006 conducted a study aimed at achieving this objective, systematically incorporating all significant findings from the inception of research in the biology of tooth movement. The study emphasizes recent advancements in cellular, molecular, tissue, and genetic responses to the application of orthodontic force. It succinctly reviews the processes of bone, periodontal ligament, and gingival remodeling in response to orthodontic force. Additionally, this review offers insights into the biological underpinnings of various adverse effects associated with orthodontic forces.

Thiago P Garlet et al.[29] in 2007 conducted a study examining the expression patterns of mRNA encoding various pro-inflammatory and anti-inflammatory cytokines in relation to extracellular matrix and bone remodeling markers. This investigation focused on the tension (T) and compression (C) sides of the periodontal ligament (PDL) in human teeth undergoing rapid maxillary expansion. The PDL of normal teeth served as a control. The findings indicate a differential expression of pro-inflammatory and anti-inflammatory cytokines in the compressed and stretched PDL during orthodontic tooth movement.

T J Fischer[30] in 2007 conducted an evaluation of the efficacy of a novel surgical technique for the treatment of palatally impacted canines. Upon completion of tooth movement, statistical analyses of the two methods indicated a reduction in treatment duration by 28-33% for canines assisted by corticotomy. No significant differences were observed in the final periodontal condition between the canines exposed using these two methods.

Mohammed Youssef et al.[31] in 2008 conducted a study to evaluate the impact of a low-level (GaAlAs) diode laser (809 nm, 100 mW) on canine retraction during orthodontic movement and to assess the associated pain levels. The findings indicate that low-level laser therapy significantly accelerates tooth movement during orthodontic treatment and effectively reduces pain levels.

Makoto Nishimura et al.[32] in 2008 states that resonance vibration significantly accelerates orthodontic tooth movement in rats by enhancing RANKL expression without additional tissue damage; study involved 6 rats per group over 21 days.

Dong Hwan Kim et al.[33] in 2008 examined whether exogenous electric current to alveolar bone could enhance orthodontic tooth movement in humans. The study included 7 female orthodontic patients. A maxillary electric appliance provided 20 µA direct current, with one maxillary canine as experimental (orthodontic force plus electric current) and the contralateral side as control (orthodontic force only). Electric current was applied for 5 hours daily, and canine movement was measured weekly. The experimental side showed 30% greater tooth movement over 4 weeks compared to the control side, with statistical significance. Movement was greater in the first two weeks for the experimental side, while the control side showed gradually decreasing movement. Results indicated that exogenous electric current might accelerate orthodontic tooth movement by one third, potentially reducing treatment duration.

Kevin G Murphy et al.[34] in 2009 states with increasing adult patients in orthodontic clinics, professionals seek ways to accelerate tooth movement. Surgical intervention affecting alveolar housing and tooth movement has been practiced for over a century. Periodontal accelerated osteogenic orthodontics (PAOO) combines selective alveolar corticotomy, particulate bone grafting, and orthodontic forces, based on the regional acceleratory phenomenon (RAP). PAOO increases alveolar bone width, reduces treatment time, improves stability, and decreases root resorption. This enhancement leads to a more intact periodontium, reduced extractions, improved facial remodeling and bone support, enhancing gingival and facial esthetics. This study aimed to describe the history, biology, procedures, indications, contraindications and complications of PAOO.

Su-Jung Kim et al.[35] in 2009 conducted a study to examine the combined effects of corticision and low-level laser therapy (LLLT) on the rate of tooth movement and paradental remodeling in beagles. The study found that periodic application of LLLT following corticision around a moving tooth resulted in a decrease in both the rate of tooth movement and alveolar remodeling activity.

M Yamaguchi[36] in 2009 presented findings on orthodontic tooth movement induced by mechanical stimuli, which is facilitated by the remodeling of the periodontal ligament (PDL) and alveolar bone. It was observed that the concentrations of RANKL in gingival crevicular fluid (GCF) increased during orthodontic tooth movement, and the ratio of RANKL to OPG concentrations in the GCF was significantly higher than in control sites. In vivo studies have demonstrated the presence of RANKL and RANK in periodontal tissues during experimental tooth movement in rat molars, indicating that PDL cells under mechanical stress may induce osteoclastogenesis through the upregulation of RANKL expression during orthodontic tooth movement.

Masaru Yamaguchi et al.[37]in 2010 reported that low-energy laser irradiation stimulated tooth movement via receptor activator of nuclear factor kappa B (RANK)/RANK ligand and macrophage colony stimulating factor/its receptor (c-Fms) systems. Matrix metalloproteinase (MMP)-9, cathepsin K, and alpha(v) beta(3) [α(v)β3] integrin are essential for osteoclastogenesis. This study examined the effects of low-energy laser irradiation on their expression during experimental tooth movement. Fifty male Wistar rats were used, with 10g force applied to molars. A Ga-Al-As diode laser irradiated the area around the moving tooth. After 7 days, tooth movement was measured using plaster models of maxillae, scanned with a 3-D measurement apparatus. Immunohistochemical staining for MMP-9, cathepsin K, and integrin subunits of α(v)β3 was performed. Intergroup comparisons used Mann-Whitney U-test for tooth movement and number of tartrate-resistant acid phosphatase (TRAP), MMP-9, cathepsin K, and α(v)β3 - positive cells. The laser irradiated group showed significantly greater tooth movement than the non-irradiated group (P < 0.05). Cells positively stained with TRAP, MMP-9, cathepsin K, and α(v)β3 increased significantly in the irradiated group on days 2-7 (P < 0.05). These findings suggest laser irradiation facilitates tooth movement velocity and expression of MMP-9, cathepsin K, and α(v)β3 in rats.

Ali H Hassan et al.[38] in 2010 stated corticotomy assisted orthodontic treatment is an efficient technique studied in recent publications. It has gained popularity as an adjunct treatment option for adult orthodontics. It involves selective alveolar decortication performed around teeth to be moved, inducing increased tissue turnover and transient osteopenia, followed by faster orthodontic tooth movement. This technique offers advantages including faster tooth movement, shorter treatment time, safer arch expansion, enhanced stability and extended envelope of tooth movement.

Shadw Mohammed Badr El-Din Aboul-Ela et al.[39] in 201 conducted a clinical evaluation of miniscrew implant-supported maxillary canine retraction facilitated by corticotomy in orthodontics. The findings indicated that the average daily rate of canine retraction was significantly higher on the corticotomy side, being twice that of the control side during the initial two months post-surgery. This rate of tooth movement decreased to 1.6 times higher in the third month and 1.06 times higher by the conclusion of the fourth month. Importantly, no molar anchorage loss was observed during canine retraction on either the operated or non-operated side. Furthermore, there were no statistically significant differences between preoperative and postoperative measurements concerning plaque index, probing depth, attachment loss, and gingival recession. The study suggests that corticotomy-facilitated orthodontics may be a viable treatment option for adults seeking orthodontic treatment with reduced treatment durations.

Hong-Suk Kim et al.[40] in 2011 introduced Speedy Surgical Orthodontics (SSO), a novel orthodontic technique that employs orthopedic forces in conjunction with temporary skeletal anchorage devices following perisegmental corticotomy to facilitate the movement of targeted dental segments. Their study examined the biological impacts of SSO on dental and periodontal structures. The findings revealed that Group II experienced significantly faster retraction and a greater amount of retraction compared to Group I. Notably, Group II did not exhibit any root resorption despite the extensive retraction, whereas Group I displayed significant root surface irregularities. Furthermore, Scanning Electron Microscopy (SEM) analysis identified multiple resorption lacunae in Group I, which were absent in Group II. The authors concluded that SSO represents an effective and advantageous orthodontic strategy for substantial en masse retraction of the maxillary anterior teeth.

Patricia J. Brooks et al.[41] in 2011 observed that monocytes may differentiate into preosteoclasts prior to their recruitment to the periodontal ligament (PDL) during the lag phase of tooth movement, with a subsequent influx of multinucleated osteoclasts occurring after six days. It was determined that a lower dose of macrophage colony-stimulating factor (M-CSF) was most effective in enhancing the extent of tooth movement and the expression of M-CSF downstream genes and tartrate-resistant acid phosphatase (TRAP), an osteoclast marker. Conversely, the administration of a higher dose of M-CSF led to a reduction in the expression of a gene downstream of M-CSF and potentially inhibited osteoclast formation. The exogenous administration of optimal dosages of M-CSF to orthodontically moved teeth presents potential for clinical studies aimed at accelerating tooth movement.

S Susan Baloul et al.[42] in 2011 conducted a study examining the role of corticotomy induced osteoclastogenesis and bone remodeling in orthodontic tooth movement, as well as the impact of selective alveolar decortication on the rate of tooth movement. The findings indicate that alveolar decortication accelerates tooth movement during the initial phase of tooth displacement. This acceleration is attributed to a coupled mechanism of bone resorption and formation during the early stages of treatment, which facilitates rapid orthodontic tooth movement.

Chung H Kau[43] in 2011 conducted a study to evaluate whether a novel device, when used in conjunction with orthodontic treatment, resulted in root resorption as observed in three-dimensional images generated by a new cone beam computerized tomography. The study found no statistically significant changes in root length from the beginning to the end of treatment when utilizing this novel robotic device. Additionally, no significant differences were observed between the roots of anterior and posterior teeth. Furthermore, no clinically significant changes in root lengths exceeding 0.5 mm were noted.

Gauri Doshi-Mehta et al.[44] in 2012conducted a study to assess the efficacy of low-intensity laser therapy in reducing the duration of orthodontic treatment and associated pain. The study observed an average increase of 30% in the rate of tooth movement with the application of low-intensity laser therapy. Additionally, pain scores on the experimental sides were significantly lower compared to the control sides.

Susan P McGorray et al.[45] in 2012 proposed that the human hormone relaxin may enhance the rate of movement and stability through its influence on the periodontal ligament. This study aimed to compare the effects of relaxin and a placebo on tooth movement and stability in human subjects. The findings indicated no significant differences in tooth movement over an 8-week treatment period or in relapse at 4 weeks post-treatment between subjects receiving weekly relaxin injections and those receiving a placebo. In both cohorts, less than half of the anticipated tooth movement was achieved after 8 weeks of treatment. It is possible that the local doses of relaxin were insufficient to impact tooth movement or short-term relapse.

Eatemad A Shoreibah et al.[46] in 2012 conducted a study with 20 adult orthodontic patients with moderate crowding of lower anterior teeth were divided into two groups: corticotomy-facilitated orthodontic movement (Group I) and conventional orthodontic therapy (Group II). Treatment time was measured from orthodontic appliance activation post-corticotomy to debracketing. Clinical periodontal parameters and periapical radiographs were recorded at baseline, post-treatment, and six months post-operatively, measuring root length and bone density. Results indicate corticotomy-facilitated orthodontic movement using the modified technique significantly reduces treatment time and decreases root resorption and adverse effects on teeth investing tissues. The acceleration of tooth movement through this technique improved patient cooperation.

Hu Long et al.[4] in 2013 conducted a study to assess the efficacy of various interventions aimed at accelerating orthodontic tooth movement. The study ultimately included nine eligible studies, examining five specific interventions: low-level laser therapy, corticotomy, electrical current, pulsed electromagnetic fields, and dentoalveolar or periodontal distraction. Six outcomes were evaluated across these studies, namely, cumulative moved distance or movement rate, time required to move the tooth to its destination, anchorage loss, periodontal health, pulp vitality, and root resorption. The researchers concluded that among the five interventions, corticotomy was found to be both effective and safe for accelerating orthodontic tooth movement. In contrast, low-level laser therapy did not demonstrate efficacy in this regard. The current evidence does not conclusively determine the effectiveness of electrical current and pulsed electromagnetic fields in accelerating orthodontic tooth movement. Dentoalveolar or periodontal distraction appears promising for accelerating orthodontic tooth movement, although it lacks robust evidence.

Su-Jung Kim et al.[47] in 2013 conducted a study to examine the effects of low-intensity laser therapy (LILT) on the remodeling of the periodontal ligament (PDL) during the phases of relapse and retention following the completion of orthodontic movement. The findings suggest that LILT influences post-orthodontic treatment stability differently, depending on whether an additional retainer is used. Specifically, when LILT is applied in conjunction with a retainer on the repositioned teeth, it may expedite the retention period by accelerating periodontal remodeling in the new tooth position. Conversely, the application of LILT on teeth without a retainer may increase the rate of relapse after treatment.

Ghada Nimeri et al.[48] in 2013 identified an increasing trend in research focused on accelerating methods for tooth movement, driven by the substantial demand among adults for reduced orthodontic treatment durations. Prolonged orthodontic treatment is associated with several disadvantages, including an elevated risk of caries, gingival recession, and root resorption. Consequently, there is a heightened demand to identify optimal methods for enhancing tooth movement while minimizing adverse effects. This study aims to examine successful approaches to tooth movement and to highlight the latest techniques in this area. The piezocision technique is regarded as one of the most effective surgical approaches due to its favorable periodontal tissue response and excellent aesthetic outcomes. Given the advantages and disadvantages associated with each approach, further research is warranted to determine the most effective method for accelerating tooth movement.

Chung How Kau et al.[49] in 2013 conducted a study to determine whether photobiomodulation reduces the duration of the alignment phase in orthodontic treatment. The findings indicated that photobiomodulation resulted in clinically significant changes in the rate of tooth movement compared to the control group during this phase of treatment.

Jorge Jofre et al.[50] in 2013 reported on three cases treated using a novel, flapless approach for minimally invasive rapid orthodontic (MIRO) procedures. This technique involves radiographic-guided micro incisions and localized piezoelectric corticotomies. The clinical implications of this method are examined herein. MIRO has been shown to reduce orthodontic treatment duration while avoiding the adverse effects commonly associated with accelerated orthodontics.

Elif I Keser et al.[51] in 2013 introduced piezocision-assisted orthodontic treatment as an innovative, minimally invasive surgical technique aimed at facilitating rapid orthodontic tooth movement. This procedure involves creating microsurgical interproximal openings in the buccal gingivae, allowing a piezoelectric knife to induce bone injury, which results in transient demineralization and subsequently accelerates tooth movement. Initially, the technique involved simultaneous incisions in both the maxilla and mandible. However, recent advancements have led to a more staged approach, wherein selected areas or segments of the arch are demineralized at different intervals during orthodontic treatment to achieve specific outcomes.

Ghizlane Genc et al.[52] in 2013 conducted a study evaluating effects of low-level laser therapy (LLLT) on orthodontic tooth movement velocity and nitric oxide levels in gingival crevicular fluid (GCF). Twenty patients (14 girls, six boys) had maxillary first premolars extracted and canines distalized. A gallium-aluminum-arsenide (Ga-Al-As) diode laser was applied on days 0, 3, 7, 14, 21, and 28 during maxillary lateral incisors retraction. Right maxillary lateral incisors formed the laser group, left ones served as control. The laser group received ten doses: five buccal and five palatal (two cervical, one middle, two apical) with 20 mW output power and 0.71 J/cm(2) dose. GCF samples were collected on mentioned days for nitric oxide analysis. Statistical analysis used Bonferroni and repeated measures variant tests ($p \leq 0.05$). LLLT accelerated orthodontic tooth movement significantly, with no significant changes in GCF nitric oxide levels during treatment.

Giuseppe Coscia et al.[53] in 2013 conducted a study evaluating mandibular anterior ridge changes using cone-beam computed tomography after augmented corticotomy with accelerated orthodontia in skeletal Class III patients. Fourteen patients with skeletal Class III were treated before orthognathic surgery using corticotomy, bone grafting, and accelerated orthodontic forces. Cone-beam computed tomograms were taken before treatment (T0) and after presurgical orthodontic treatment (T1). Vertical alveolar bone changes and horizontal bone thickness were measured at mandibular incisors. Patients showed significant proclination at T1. Alveolar bone thickness increased buccally at midroot and apex levels, showing significant labial augmentation (P < .05). Vertical bone change showed no significant loss. The technique provided adequate incisor decompensation by increasing labial bone thickness without vertical bone loss, reducing periodontal complications associated with traditional orthodontics.

I Ize-Iyamu et al.[54] in 2013 a randomized clinical study observed that diode laser procedures necessitated infiltration anesthesia in only 16.7% of cases, in contrast to 90.9% in conventional surgery ($P<0.001$). The laser technique consistently demonstrated statistically significant advantages, including a substantial reduction in postoperative pain, minimal bleeding, the elimination of suture requirements, and comparable treatment durations. Patients reported enhanced postoperative comfort and healing. Although this constitutes a single study, the comprehensive statistical analysis, conducted at a 95% confidence level, provides robust evidence supporting the laser's potential as a superior surgical technique in orthodontic soft tissue management.

Shailesh Shenava et al.[3] in 2014 reviewed that orthodontic treatment duration is the primary patient concern. Long treatment time increases risks of dental caries, gingival recession and root resorption, creating demand for faster tooth movement methods with minimal disadvantages. Orthodontic treatment works by delivering force to a tooth and adjacent tissues, triggering mechanical, chemical, and cellular events that enable tooth movement. This process typically takes 12-48 months. To accelerate tooth movement, various methods are available including surgical procedures (corticotomy, piezosurgery), mechanical stimulation (vibration, lasers), drugs, and magnets. These methods have reduced treatment times by up to 70%. This article reviews the latest methods to accelerate orthodontic tooth movement.

Zana Kalajzic et al.[55] in 2014 conducted a study to examine the impact of externally applied cyclical (vibratory) forces on the rate of tooth movement, the structural integrity of the periodontal ligament, and alveolar bone remodeling. Their findings indicated that cyclical forces significantly inhibited tooth movement. Histological analysis revealed notable disorganization of the collagen fibril structure within the periodontal ligament during tooth movement. Additionally, tooth movement resulted in a significant increase in osteoclast parameters on the compression side of the alveolar bone and a significant decrease in bone volume fraction in the molar region compared to controls. Consequently, they concluded that the application of cyclical forces significantly inhibited tooth movement.

H Cao et al.[56] in 2014 conducted a study which presents compelling evidence that mechanical compressive force induces Adrb2 expression in periodontal ligament cells. Experimental findings in rat models revealed that activation of Adrb2 significantly enhanced orthodontic tooth movement, increasing it from 300 to 540 μm after seven days of force application. Mechanistically, the researchers determined that mechanical force upregulates Adrb2, elevates the RANKL/OPG ratio, and facilitates osteoclast differentiation. Notably, Adrb1/2-/- mice exhibited a markedly reduced tooth movement (19.5 μm) compared to wild-type mice (107.6 μm), thereby conclusively associating Adrb2 with the acceleration of tooth movement.

Preeti Bhattacharya et al.[57] in 2014 found significant differences between corticotomy and conventional orthodontic techniques. The ct study showed reduced retraction time (p<0.001) and changes in alveolar bone thickness, with significant differences in total alveolar thickness at the crest region for all incisors (p<0.05), and at mid-root and apical levels for specific teeth (p<0.05). The research demonstrates that corticotomies accelerate orthodontic treatment while increasing alveolar width, suggesting value for adult orthodontic patients seeking efficient treatment.

Chidchanok Leethanakul et al.[58] in 2014 conducted a split-mouth study involving 18 female participants, wherein it was observed that the surgical reduction of interseptal bone thickness, when combined with conventional orthodontic appliances, resulted in an increase in canine movement from 3.4 mm to 5.4 mm (P = .002). Although this technique demonstrated a statistically significant enhancement in mesio-distal movement, no significant differences were observed in canine angulation or rotation. The researchers concluded that this surgical approach can facilitate tooth movement when interseptal bone is adequately reduced, presenting a promising minimal-trauma method to potentially expedite orthodontic treatment. Interseptal bone reduction can significantly accelerate maxillary canine retraction by approximately 2 mm over a period of 3 months.

M Alikhani et al.[59] in 2015 demonstrated that micro-osteoperforations (MOPs) represent a minimally invasive technique capable of significantly accelerating orthodontic tooth movement by inducing controlled inflammatory responses. The research provides substantial evidence from both animal and human studies, indicating that MOPs increase the rate of tooth movement by 2.3-fold, accompanied by notable elevations in inflammatory markers. These findings have been corroborated in both rat models and human subjects, revealing enhanced canine retraction rates without additional pain or discomfort for patients.

Jabir Ahamed Arakkal et al.[60] in 2015 said corticotomy assisted orthodontic treatment involves selective alveolar decortication through lines and grooves around teeth intended for orthodontic movement. This procedure induces increased bone turnover, enabling faster tooth movement. The technique offers advantages including accelerated tooth movement, reduced treatment time, safer arch expansion, enhanced stability and extended movement envelope.

Dubravko Pavlin et al.[61] in 2015 conducted a parallel, double-blind, randomized controlled trial assessing the effect of low-level cyclic loading on orthodontic tooth movement rate. The study included 45 orthodontic patients with fixed appliances at UTHSC San Antonio Orthodontic Department, requiring maxillary first premolar extraction and posterior anchorage. Subjects were randomized into vibration (n=23) and control (n=22) groups using computer-generated scheduling, with all participants blinded to assignment. The vibration group received cyclic loading for 20 min/day via AcceleDent device (0.25 N force at 30 Hz), while controls used a non-vibrating device. Analysis of monthly maxillary canine retraction showed significantly higher movement rate in the AcceleDent group at 1.16 mm/month (95% CI: 0.86–1.46) versus 0.79 mm/month (95% CI: 0.49–1.09) in controls, with 0.37 mm/month difference (95% CI: 0.07–0.81, P = 0.05). Results demonstrated that cyclic loading at 0.25 N/30 Hz increases tooth movement rate during orthodontic treatment.

JiaQi Wu et al.[62] in 2015 undertook a study to evaluate the efficacy of the improved accelerated osteogenic orthodontic (IAOO) procedure in reducing the duration of preoperative orthodontic treatment for patients requiring Class III surgical intervention. The research also sought to investigate the influence of the IAOO procedure on the pattern of tooth movement during the closure of extraction spaces. The results demonstrated that the IAOO procedure can decrease the duration of surgical orthodontic treatment for skeletal Class III patients by an average of over six months. Nonetheless, the IAOO procedures do not contribute to the preservation of anchorage.

Chi-Yang Tsai et al.[63] in 2016 investigated the impact of flapless micro-osteoperforation and corticision on the rate of orthodontic tooth movement in rats. Their findings indicated that these two minimally invasive flapless surgical techniques enhanced bone remodeling and osteoclast activity, thereby accelerating orthodontic tooth movement for a duration of at least two weeks in rats. The study observed no significant differences in outcomes between flapless micro-osteoperforation and corticision in the rats.

Sertac Aksakalli et al.[64] in 2016 compared canine distalization and transversal changes using pre- and post-distalization dental casts scanned with an orthodontic scanner. The gingival indices and mobility scores were calculated. Three-dimensional analysis showed significant differences in tooth movement with lesser anchorage loss and greater canine distalization. The distalization time was shortened in the experimental group. Piezocision-assisted distalization accelerates tooth movement, reduces anchorage loss for posterior teeth, does not cause maxillary transversal changes, and has no adverse effects on periodontal health.

Chidchanok Leethanakul et al.[65] in 2016 studied the impact of vibratory stimuli on interleukin (IL)-1β secretion during maxillary canine distalization. Using a split-mouth design with 15 participants, bilateral maxillary first premolar extractions were followed by canine distalization. The experimental side received 60 g of force for three months plus vibratory stimuli via electric toothbrush for 15 minutes daily over two months, while the control side received only orthodontic force. Gingival crevicular fluid (GCF) was collected monthly from both canines‘ mesial and distal aspects. IL-1β levels were measured using enzyme-linked immunosorbent assay, and canine movement was tracked monthly. Results showed that vibratory stimuli with light orthodontic force enhanced IL-1β secretion in GCF and accelerated tooth movement.

Eric J. W. Liou[66] in 2016 stated surgical-assisted accelerated orthodontic tooth movement is most effective, but its disadvantages include bone surgery and alveolar bone loss that undermines periodontal support. Submucosal injection of platelet rich plasma (PRP) accelerates orthodontic tooth movement by simulating bone insult effects without surgery. They revealed PRP injection accelerated mandibular or maxillary alignment 1.7 folds faster, with acceleration being dose-dependent when PRP fold was <12.5. The optimal PRP fold for >2-fold acceleration ranged from 9.5 to 12.5. The injection of PRP on the pressure side of en masse anterior retraction decreased 71-77% of alveolar bone loss dose-dependently, with no bone loss when PRP fold exceeded 11.0. The optimal PRP fold for best performance in acceleration and alveolar bone preservation is 11.0-12.5.

Young Guk Park[67] in 2016 states orthodontic tooth movement occurs when forces applied to teeth evoke cellular responses in surrounding tissues, including periodontal ligament, alveolar bone and gingiva. Understanding biological events during tooth movement is crucial for orthodontists, as these processes vary between individuals due to differences in periodontal metabolism and bone density. Orthodontics integrates mechanics and biology in unique physiological systems. These variations explain differences in treatment outcomes between patients with similar malocclusions treated identically. Clinical trials have explored methods to facilitate tooth movement through biomechanical, pharmaceutical, surgical, electrical, or tissue engineering approaches. 'Corticision', a minimally invasive procedure without flap elevation, accelerates tooth movement through enhanced structural turnover. This article presents the procedure's technical aspects and biological basis for accelerated treatment.

Konstantinia Almpani et al.[68] in 2016 stated surgical techniques for accelerating orthodontic tooth movement have been tested for over 100 years. Since original methods were extremely invasive and associated with tooth morbidity, research in this field followed an episodic trend. Modern approaches represent a refined strategy where only cortical plate around orthodontic tooth movement is desired, abandoning the bony block concept. Selective alveolar decortication has been a reproducible gold standard, with its mechanism being the induction of rapid tooth movement through periodontal ligament involvement. Recent techniques include less invasive procedures like piezoelectricity and corticision. This article focused on the evolution of surgical approaches and mechanistic concepts underlying surgically accelerated orthodontic tooth movements.

Noha Hussein Abbas et al.[69] in 2016 said that application of corticotomy and piezocision techniques has been shown to expedite canine retraction in orthodontic treatment, yielding modest yet statistically significant enhancements in the rate of tooth movement. In a rct study involving 20 patients aged 15 to 25, it was observed that surgical interventions resulted in increased rates of canine movement compared to conventional methods. Specifically, corticotomies demonstrated superior canine movement rates at four distinct time points, with mean canine crown tip movements of 1.22 mm (±0.08 mm) in the corticotomy group and 0.99 mm (±0.1 mm) in the piezocision group over a 12-week period.

C. Charavet et al.[70] in 2016 conducted a randomized controlled trial having 24 adult patients with mild dental overcrowding were allocated into two groups: conventional orthodontics and piezocision. The piezocision group exhibited a notable 43% reduction in overall treatment duration compared to the control group. Importantly, periodontal parameters remained stable, and no increase in root resorption was detected. Patient satisfaction was significantly higher in the piezocision group, although 50% of patients experienced minor scarring. This study provides compelling evidence supporting piezocision as a minimally invasive technique to expedite orthodontic tooth movement, with the consideration that patients with high smile lines should be cautious due to the potential risk of scarring.

Tracy Cheung et al.[71] in 2016 conducted an experimental study by positioning five micro-osteoperforations (MOPs) around the maxillary first molars in rats to assess tooth movement outcomes. The side with MOPs exhibited a 1.86-fold increase in the rate of tooth movement, decreased bone density around the first molars, increased osteoclast numbers, and new bone formation. Importantly, three-dimensional volumetric analysis of all five roots revealed no statistically significant differences in root volumes, indicating that the technique does not compromise root integrity. The researchers concluded that MOPs may provide a readily available and efficient method to reduce orthodontic treatment time with enhanced patient acceptance.

Timothy Shaughnessy et al.[72] in 2016 did an investigation involving 19 orthodontic patients revealed that daily photobiomodulation (PBM) treatment enhanced the average rate of tooth movement from 0.44 mm/week to 1.27 mm/week, representing a 2.9-fold increase. Patients utilizing the PBM device achieved dental alignment in an average of 48 days, in contrast to 104 days for the control group. The results were statistically significant (p = 0.0002 for movement rate, p = 0.0053 for treatment duration), with a 93% compliance rate among patients for daily treatments. Intraoral PBM significantly accelerates orthodontic tooth alignment, reducing treatment duration by 54% in this preliminary clinical study.

Francisco Muñoz et al.[73] in 2016 conducted a pilot study of 11 patients, post-surgical pain was "mild" (45.5%) or "moderate" (54.5%), with post-surgical inflammation being "mild" (89.9%) or "moderate" (9.1%). Inflammation resolution began by day 4 and completed by day 8 in all patients. The study shows that leukocyte and Platelet-Rich Fibrin (L-PRF) provides clinical benefits in reducing post-surgical pain and inflammation during Periodontally Accelerated Osteogenic Orthodontics (PAOO). However, the limited sample size and single-center design limit result generalizability. The orthodontic treatment averaged 9.3 months, with cases remaining stable over 2 years.

Mohammad Moaffak A AlSayed Hasan et al.[74] in 2017 conducted a study involving 26 patients divided into laser and control groups, with LLLT applied using an 830-nm wavelength laser at tooth roots. Results showed significant differences between groups, with LLLT reducing treatment time (P < .001) and improving alignment (P = .004 and P = .001). The laser was applied after archwire insertion and repeated regularly, demonstrating effectiveness in accelerating orthodontic tooth movement in patients with maxillary incisor crowding.

Alaa M H Alfawal et al.[75] in 2018 conducted a single-center randomized controlled trial with 36 Class II division I patients (aged 15-27), researchers found significant acceleration of tooth movement using Piezocision and laser-assisted flapless corticotomy techniques. The split-mouth study with 17 patients per group showed greater canine retraction rates in experimental versus control sides (p < 0.001), with overall retraction duration reduced by 25% (p ≤ 0.001). No significant differences were found in anchorage loss or canine rotation, indicating both techniques effectively accelerate orthodontic tooth movement. Piezocision and laser-assisted flapless corticotomy accelerate canine retraction by two-fold in the first month and 1.5-fold in the second month.

Sonal Attri et al.[76] in 2018 conducted a randomized controlled trial by involving 60 patients, it was found that micro-osteoperforations (MOP) performed distal to the canines every 28 days significantly increased the rate of tooth movement (p<0.05). The experimental group received MOP in conjunction with fixed appliances, whereas the control group utilized identical brackets without MOP. The study conclusively demonstrates that MOP can enhance the efficiency of orthodontic tooth movement without compromising patient comfort or increasing pain perception.

A P S Gil et al.[77] in 2018 conducted a systematic review and concluded that corticotomy-facilitated orthodontics results in accelerated tooth movement with minimal complications, such as pain and swelling. Nevertheless, the methodological quality of the existing studies was found to be low, offering only low to moderate scientific evidence. Alveolar corticotomies have the potential to significantly reduce the duration of orthodontic treatment, with the mean treatment time decreasing from 16.4 months to 8.85 months.

Alissa Maria Varella et al.[78] in 2018 conducted a split-mouth study involving 10 participants aged 14-25, the application of a gallium-aluminum-arsenide diode laser (940 nm, 8 J/cm^2) to experimental canines resulted in elevated IL-1β levels compared to control canines. The experimental canines exhibited a significant increase in IL-1β levels ($P < 0.001$) and demonstrated tooth movement ranging from 4.450 to 4.4903 mm, in contrast to the control canines, which showed movement between 2.025 and 2.0501 mm. The study established a correlation between IL-1β levels and tooth movement. Low-level laser therapy (LLLT) was found to enhance IL-1β levels and expedite orthodontic tooth movement.

Saritha Sivarajan et al.[79] in 2019 conducted a split-mouth randomized clinical trial in which mean canine retraction was 4.16 mm with micro-osteoperforation (MOP) versus 3.06 mm without MOP. MOP frequency groups showed increased distalization: 0.89 mm (4-weekly), 1.08 mm (8-weekly), and 1.33 mm (12-weekly) compared to control, with p-values from .01 to .002. The authors deemed the difference "unlikely to be clinically significant." Subjects reported pain, with 60% rating it moderate and 15% severe, affecting chewing and speech. While MOP significantly accelerates mini-implant supported canine retraction, its clinical impact appears minimal.

Amira A Aboalnaga et al.[80] in 2019 conducted a primary split-mouth randomized controlled trial involving 18 patients, no statistically significant difference was observed in the overall rate of canine retraction, which was measured at 0.99 ± 0.3 mm per month. However, the total distances moved by the canine center and apex were significantly greater on the micro-osteoperforation (MOP) side compared to the control side, with mean differences of 0.37 ± 0.63 mm (P < 0.05) and 0.47 ± 0.56 mm (P < 0.01), respectively. The study noted significantly greater movement at the canine center and apex in MOP sites. While MOPs do not consistently accelerate the rate of canine retraction, they may facilitate root movement.

Neda Babanouri et al.[81] in 2020 conducted a single-center, split-mouth, triple-blind randomized trial researchers studied two MOP approaches: one with 3 buccal perforations and another with 3 buccal and 3 palatal perforations. The study included 28 patients aged 16.3 to 35.2 years undergoing orthodontic treatment. Statistically significant difference in canine retraction rate between MOP groups and control sides noted. Increasing perforation numbers significantly accelerated canine retraction. However, the authors noted the acceleration was not clinically significant.

Kanchan Prafulla Narkhede et al.[82] in 2021 did a systematic review which analyzed eight studies (six animal and two human), finding that three animal studies and one human randomized controlled trial reported PRP increased tooth movement rate when used as an orthodontic treatment adjunct.

Wasundhara Ashok Bhad Patil et al.[83] in 2022 conducted a randomized split-mouth design involving 19 patients. A device generating pulsed electromagnetic fields (PEMF) was incorporated into a removable appliance, which patients wore for 8-10 hours during the canine retraction phase. The experimental side was subjected to PEMF exposure. Although the findings are promising, the limited sample size and the study's singular nature indicate the necessity for more extensive research to conclusively determine the efficacy of PEMF in reducing the duration of orthodontic treatment. PEMF therapy demonstrates potential in expediting orthodontic tooth movement, as evidenced by a clinical investigation reporting a 31% increase in the rate of tooth movement.

Giuseppa Bilello et al.[84] in 2022 conducted a clinical trial by patients using AcceleDent vibratory device with a 7-day aligner protocol which completed treatment faster than the 14-day protocol. Patients using AcceleDent averaged 9.0 ± 1.0 days per aligner, versus 15.4 ± 1.2 days in controls (P < 0.001). The vibration group experienced reduced pain during the first week (P < 0.05). While this study had 24 participants, results suggest potential for accelerating aligner treatments. Low-frequency vibration can significantly reduce aligner treatment duration and improve patient comfort during orthodontic treatment.

Yaman Guray et al.[85] in 2023 evaluated light-emitting photobiomodulation therapy's (LPT) effect on canine distalization rate in 60 extraction spaces from upper first premolars of 30 patients (15 LPT, 15 control). PG-segmented canine retraction springs were used. The LPT group received Biolux OrthoPulse treatment (850 nm LED light, 63 mW/cm). Mean distalization rates were 1.36 mm/21 days in LPT and 1.02 mm/21 days in control groups, showing statistical significance (p < 0.001). Anchorage loss, canine rotations, and molar inclinations showed no significant differences between groups. LPT accelerated orthodontic tooth movement by 33%.

Rashad I Shaadouh et al.[86] in 2024 conducted a randomized controlled trial with 38 participants, which demonstrated that the rate of en-masse retraction was significantly higher in the low-intensity electrical stimulation (LIES) group compared to the traditional retraction method (1.02±0.08 mm/month vs. 0.73±0.04 mm/month; P<0.001). The application of LIES modestly accelerated the retraction of upper anterior teeth by approximately 28% in young adult patients with Class II division 1 malocclusion.

Mudar M Mousa et al.[87] in 2025 demonstrated that the primary randomized controlled trial of the group receiving both low-level laser therapy (LLLT) and piezocision achieved the highest retraction rate, measuring 1.32 ± 0.19 mm/month. This rate surpasses the 1.09 ± 0.13 mm/month observed with piezocision alone and the 0.75 ± 0.06 mm/month associated with conventional methods. The combination of LLLT and piezocision significantly enhances the en-masse retraction of upper anterior teeth, achieving an acceleration of up to 43.8% compared to conventional techniques.

CHAPTER III

METHODS OF ACCELERATING TOOTH MOVEMENT

There are three phases of tooth movement: the initial phase, which is characterized by rapid movement after the application of force; followed by a lag period, where little or no movement, and the last, postlag phase, where gradual or sudden increase of movement occurs [88].

Initial phase	Rapid movement after application of force
Lag phase	Little or no movement
Final phase	Gradual or sudden increase of movement

The initial stage of tooth movement is characterized by acute inflammatory responses, during which leukocytes migrate from blood capillaries and produce cytokines. This process stimulates the secretion of prostaglandins and growth factors [29].

The acute phase is succeeded by the chronic phase, characterized by the proliferation of fibroblasts, endothelial cells, osteoblasts, and alveolar bone marrow cells, which are involved in the remodeling process [28].

METHODS TO EXPEDITE ORTHODONTIC TOOTH MOVEMENT CAN BE BROADLY CATEGORIZED INTO THE FOLLOWING APPROACHES

A) Biological Approach,

B) Device-Assisted Approach,

C) Surgical Approach.

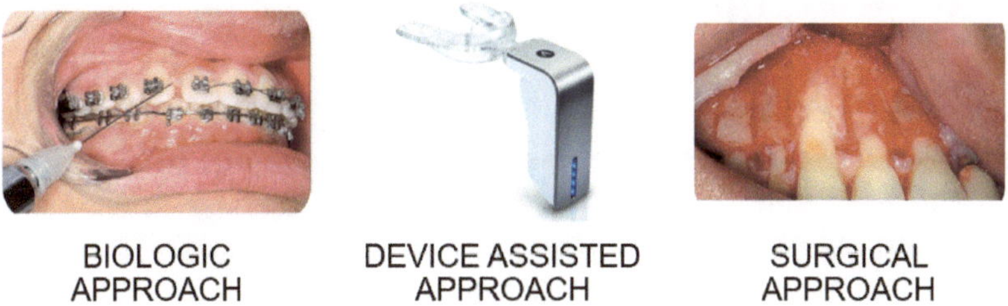

FIG 1: Methods of accelerating tooth movement

CHAPTER IV

BIOLOGICAL APPROACH

Numerous pharmacological agents have been employed historically to expedite orthodontic tooth movement, yielding successful outcomes. These agents include vitamin D [14], prostaglandins [18], interleukins, parathyroid hormone, and misoprostol, among others [89]. Experimental studies have utilized these compounds exogenously to enhance tooth movement in humans. However, each of these drugs is associated with certain adverse effects. For instance, vitamin D, when injected into the periodontal ligament (PDL), elevates the levels of lactate dehydrogenase (LDH) and creatine phosphokinase (CPK) enzymes; prostaglandins induce a generalized inflammatory response and contribute to root resorption. Consequently, no pharmacological agent currently exists that can safely accelerate orthodontic tooth movement. Extensive research has been conducted on exogenous molecules such as prostaglandin E (PGE2), cytokines derived from lymphocytes and monocytes, receptor activator of nuclear factor kappa B ligand (RANKL), and macrophage colony-stimulating factor (MCSF) to develop methods for enhancing tooth movement in both animal models and human subjects.

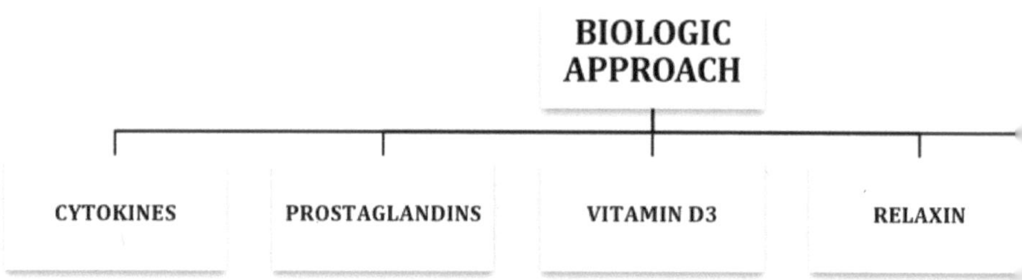

EFFECT OF CYTOKINES ON TOOTH MOVEMENT

Elevated concentrations of cytokines, including interleukins IL-1, IL-2, IL-3, IL-6, IL-8, and Tumor Necrosis Factor Alpha (TNF), have been identified as significant contributors to bone remodeling. Notably, interleukin-1 (IL-1) enhances osteoclast function via its receptor on osteoclasts [90]. Additionally, mechanical stress induced by orthodontic treatment has been shown to elevate the production of prostaglandin PGE and IL-1 beta within the periodontal ligaments. These findings were derived from experiments conducted on cats, where one canine was subjected to distal tipping with an 80 g force for varying durations, ranging from hours to days. Immunohistochemistry and microphotometry were employed to assess the intensity of PGE and IL-1 beta, which was found to be most pronounced on the tension side [11].

Orthodontic tooth movement is facilitated by the remodeling of the periodontal ligament (PDL) and alveolar bone in response to mechanical loading, a process believed to be mediated by various host mediators, such as cytokines. Utilizing real-time polymerase chain reaction (PCR), we examined the expression patterns of mRNA encoding several pro- and anti-inflammatory cytokines in relation to various extracellular matrix and bone remodeling markers on the tension (T) and compression (C) sides of the PDL in human teeth subjected to rapid maxillary expansion. The PDL of normal teeth served as a control. The results indicated that both T and C sides exhibited significantly elevated expression of all targets compared to controls, with the exception of type I collagen (COL-I) and tissue inhibitor of metalloproteinase-1 (TIMP-1) on the C side. When comparing the C and T sides, the C side demonstrated higher expression of tumor necrosis factor-a (TNF-a), receptor activator of nuclear factor-jB ligand (RANKL), and matrix metalloproteinase-1 (MMP-1), whereas the T side showed higher expression of interleukin 10 (IL-10), TIMP-1, COL-I, osteoprotegerin (OPG), and osteocalcin (OCN). The expression of transforming growth factor-b (TGF-b) was similar on both C and T sides. Our data reveal a differential expression of pro- and anti-inflammatory cytokines in compressed and stretched PDL during orthodontic tooth movement.

Orthodontic tooth movement is facilitated through the remodeling of the periodontal ligament (PDL) and alveolar bone in response to mechanical loading. The complexity of mechanical loading patterns arises from the intricate anatomy and tissue structure, as demonstrated by recent finite element analysis. However, finite element studies are limited to determining pure mechanical force and cannot predict the biological tissue response. Despite the complexity of mechanical loading, two distinct opposing sides are identified: tension (T), where the displacement of the dental root induces a strain force in the PDL fibers, and compression (C), where a compression force is exerted by the root against the bone, resulting in the unloading of fibers. These sides are characterized by the predominant forces and the overall tissue response observed.

The transduction of mechanical forces to cells initiates a biological response, described as aseptic inflammation, mediated by various inflammatory cytokines and not indicative of a pathological condition. Unlike chronic inflammatory responses, which are sustained by persistent stimuli and lead to tissue damage, the expression of inflammatory mediators following orthodontic force application is transient and crucial for orthodontic movement, as evidenced by the ability of anti-inflammatory drugs to inhibit tooth movement. This tissue response initially involves vascular changes, followed by the synthesis of prostaglandins, cytokines, and growth factors. These mediators are believed to activate tissue remodeling, characterized by selective bone resorption or deposition in the C and T regions of the PDL, respectively. Bone formation is driven by factors such as bone morphogenetic proteins, cytokines, and growth factors, which promote the differentiation of precursor cells into the osteoblast phenotype. Orthodontic tooth movement is achieved through PDL remodeling, triggered by a force-induced biological response described as aseptic inflammation. Despite the complexity of mechanical loading patterns, two distinct opposing sides can be discerned in the periodontium—a T side and a C side—based on the direction and nature of predominant forces and overall tissue response. Tissue remodeling is modulated by pro- and anti-inflammatory cytokines and is likely influenced by distinct cytokine subsets. The pro-inflammatory cytokine, TNF- α, is present in high levels in the gingival crevicular fluid during orthodontic tooth movement and, in mice, is particularly expressed on the C side [48]. Our data demonstrate an increased expression of TNF- α in both C and T sides compared to controls.

However, the expression of TNF- α was markedly elevated on the C side, which is characterized by bone resorption activity and increased RANKL levels. TNF- α functions as a positive regulator of RANKL-mediated osteoclastogenesis, and the inhibition of TNF- α signaling results in a reduction of tartrate-resistant acid phosphatase (TRAP)-positive osteoclasts and diminished tooth movement in rodent models. Beyond the expression of genes associated with bone resorption, TNF- α also stimulates periodontal ligament (PDL) cells to produce matrix metalloproteinases (MMPs). Consistent with previous research, our findings indicate higher

MMP-1 mRNA levels on the C side compared to the T side, supporting the hypothesis that the pro-inflammatory cytokine TNF- α contributes to catabolic activity. Conversely, the roles of anti-inflammatory cytokines in orthodontic tooth movement remain inadequately understood. Our results reveal that IL-10 expression is significantly elevated on the C side compared to the T side. This observation aligns with the finding that tensile strain induces IL-10 synthesis in PDL. However, IL-10 mRNA was not detected during orthodontic tooth movement in rats via in situ hybridization. Previous studies have highlighted the significant role of IL-10 in bone metabolism in vivo, as IL-10-deficient mice exhibit decreased osteoblast generation and bone formation. Conversely, in vitro data suggest that IL-10 can suppress osteoblast differentiation in murine bone marrow cultures by inhibiting TGF- β production. However, given the high TGF- β expression on both the C and T sides, and the absence of negative correlations between IL-10 and TGF-b levels, we posit that such inhibition does not occur during tooth movement. The effect of IL-10 on osteoclasts appears more definitive, as IL-10 inhibits bone resorption through the simultaneous up-regulation of osteoprotegerin (OPG) and down-regulation of RANKL expression. Correspondingly, a positive correlation was observed between IL-10 and OPG levels, while IL-10 and RANKL levels exhibited a negative correlation. Therefore, the increased expression of IL-10 may be associated with reduced osteoclast function and heightened osteoblast activity, characteristic of the T side.

Supporting this, positive correlations were found between IL-10 and osteocalcin (OCN) levels, suggesting that IL-10 contributes to bone formation on the T side. IL-10 may also influence extracellular matrix (ECM) metabolism through opposing pathways. One possibility is that IL-10, despite inhibiting local inflammation, does not affect collagen metabolism outcomes. Alternatively, IL-10 may inhibit COL-I synthesis by down-regulating TGF- β release. As previously discussed, given the absence of any correlation between IL-10 and TGF- β levels, we believe that such inhibition does not occur in PDL cells during tooth movement.

Conversely, IL-10 may also exert an indirect influence on turnover by modulating the balance between MMPs and TIMPs. IL-10 is known to upregulate TIMPs while inhibiting MMP activity, thereby contributing to the maintenance of tissue integrity and ECM deposition. Supporting this notion, positive correlations have been observed between the levels of

IL-10, COL-I, and TIMP-1, suggesting a potential anabolic role for IL-10. Another cytokine implicated in orthodontic tooth movement is TGF-β, whose mRNA expression has been found to increase on both the compression (C) and tension (T) sides compared to controls. Consistent with this, TGF-β expression is elevated during orthodontic tooth movement, being detected in osteoblasts in the T zone and osteoclasts in the C zone, indicating a comprehensive role for this cytokine in orthodontic tooth movement. TGF-β is a pleiotropic cytokine that regulates cell growth, differentiation, and matrix production. Generally, TGF-β exhibits anabolic functions, enhancing the proliferation and chemotaxis of PDL cells and upregulating COL-I expression. TGF-β also exerts anabolic effects on bone tissue by recruiting osteoblast precursors, inducing their differentiation, and promoting the production of bone matrix proteins.

Additionally, TGF-β downregulates the transcription of pro-inflammatory mediators and several MMPs while upregulating TIMPs. Correspondingly, a positive correlation between TGF-β and TIMP-1 levels has been identified. Thus, TGF-β may exert an anabolic effect in the PDL during tooth movement, facilitating the synthesis of both soft and mineralized connective tissues on the T side. However, its expression is also elevated on the C side, which is likely characterized by resorptive activity. Typically, TGF-β is described as inhibiting the recruitment of osteoclast precursor cells and suppressing osteoclast activity, although some studies suggest that TGF-β may also play a role in bone resorption induction. Nevertheless, no correlations between TGF-β levels and bone remodeling markers have been identified. Indeed, the role of TGF-β in osteoclastogenesis and bone resorption is complex and appears to depend on cellular phenotype, stage of cell differentiation, and TGF-β concentration. It is important to note that the individual effects of cytokines on bone and ECM metabolism are usually investigated in highly controlled systems, such as in vitro studies or knockout mice models. When interpreting in vivo data, it is essential to estimate the putative function of cytokines within a complex environment characterized by the presence of numerous cell types, cytokines, and hormones that interact and influence one another.

It is also crucial to acknowledge that mechanical loading patterns are intricate, and the tissue responses observed on the two opposing sides are likely predominantly, though not exclusively, the result of opposing forces.

Data indeed demonstrate a concomitant occurrence of TGF- β, IL-10, and TNF- α on both the T and C sides, albeit with seemingly distinct expression patterns. Although the results of the present study do not provide conclusive insights into the cause-and-effect relationships between cytokine expression and tissue response during orthodontic tooth movement, we tentatively propose that the elevated level of TGF- β expression observed on both the C and T sides represents an overall anabolic response (inducing ECM synthesis and bone formation) that can be differentially modulated by TNF- α and IL-10. The higher TNF- α expression on the C side possibly drives the predominance of catabolic activity through the up-regulation of RANKL and MMPs, which may potentially counteract the effects of TGF- β and IL-10. Conversely, the elevated levels of IL-10, TIMP, and OPG expression on the T side may result in the predominance of anabolic activities. Further studies are necessary to more fully understand the role of pro- and anti-inflammatory mediators in tissue remodeling during orthodontic tooth movement. Once differentiated, osteoblasts produce proteins such as type I collagen (COL-I), osteocalcin (OCN), and alkaline phosphatase, which are indicative of bone formation. Conversely, bone resorption is initiated by the engagement of the receptor activator of nuclear factor B (RANK), present on osteoclast precursors, with its ligand RANKL, expressed particularly on osteoblasts. The interaction between RANK and RANKL triggers the differentiation and activation of osteoclasts, an event regulated by osteoprotegerin (OPG), a decoy receptor that inhibits the RANK–RANKL interaction. Recent studies highlight the involvement of the RANK system in orthodontic tooth movement.

In addition to alveolar bone, the collagenous extracellular matrix (ECM) is also remodeled on the compressed and stretched sides of the PDL during orthodontic tooth movement. Among host proteases that target the ECM, matrix metalloproteases (MMPs; a family of zinc and calcium-dependent proteases) play a role in both the degradation and remodeling of matrix proteins during various physiological and pathological processes. MMP-1, or interstitial collagenase, is active against native triple-helical interstitial collagens and can initiate tissue remodeling.

The activation of matrix metalloproteinases (MMPs) is regulated by a group of endogenous proteins known as tissue inhibitors of metalloproteinases (TIMPs), each of which can inhibit nearly all members of the MMP family in a non-specific manner. MMPs and TIMPs are integral to the physiological turnover of periodontal tissues and are believed to play significant roles in orthodontic tooth movement. The metabolism of both soft and mineralized connective tissues can be modulated by cytokines and growth factors, suggesting their potential involvement in tissue remodeling during orthodontic tooth movement. Inflammatory cytokines, such as tumor necrosis factor-alpha (TNF- α), exhibit a predominant catabolic effect, acting as positive regulators of osteoclastogenesis and MMP expression. Conversely, transforming growth factor-beta (TGF- β) exerts an anabolic effect by inducing osteoblastogenesis and extracellular matrix (ECM) synthesis, in addition to its anti-inflammatory properties. Similarly, interleukin-10 (IL-10) also possesses anti-inflammatory properties and generally exerts an inhibitory effect that can modulate both tissue deposition and degradation. In the context of orthodontic tooth movement, TNF- α levels are found to be upregulated following the application of orthodontic force and are thought to play crucial roles in bone resorption. Indeed, studies using animal models demonstrate that the absence of TNF-α signaling results in impaired tooth movement, although the mechanisms underlying their function remain unknown.

On the other hand, the potential role of anti-inflammatory cytokines in orthodontic tooth movement has been less thoroughly explored. TGF-β expression has been observed to increase during orthodontic tooth movement on both the tension (T) and compression (C) sides, where it is believed to influence the remodeling of both soft and bone tissues. Conversely, the anti-inflammatory cytokine IL-10 was not detected during orthodontic tooth movement in rats via in situ hybridization. Recent studies suggest a differential expression of tissue remodeling mediators on the T and C sides of the periodontal ligament (PDL) throughout tooth movement. However, the balance between pro-inflammatory and anti-inflammatory mediators on the T and C sides, and their impact on PDL and bone remodeling, remain unknown [39].

The elevated concentration of cytokines, including interleukins IL-1, IL-2, IL-3, IL-6, IL-8, and tumor necrosis factor alpha (TNF), has been identified as a significant factor in bone remodeling. Notably, interleukin-1 (IL-1) enhances osteoclast function via its receptor on osteoclasts. Additionally, mechanical stresses induced by orthodontic treatment have been shown to increase the production of prostaglandin PGE and IL-1 beta in the periodontal ligament. Experiments conducted on cats, where one canine was subjected to an 80g distal force for varying durations, revealed through immunohistochemistry and microphotometry that the intensity of PGE and IL-1 beta was highest on the tension side. Other cytokines involved in the acceleration of tooth movement include RANKL, a membrane-bound protein on osteoclasts that binds to RANK on osteoclasts, promoting osteoclastogenesis. Conversely, osteoprotegerin (OPG) competes with RANKL for binding to osteoclasts, thereby inhibiting osteoclastogenesis. Bone remodeling is thus a balancc between the (RANKL-RANK) system and the OPG compound.

In this context, the utilization of biological molecules to expedite tooth movement has been evidenced in two distinct experiments[43]. These studies demonstrated that the transfer of the RANKL gene to periodontal tissue resulted in sustained gene expression, thereby enhancing osteoclastogenesis and accelerating tooth movement in rats. Conversely, the transfer of the OPG gene was found to inhibit orthodontic tooth movement [93]. In a separate study, it was observed that the movement of juvenile teeth occurs at a faster rate compared to that of adults. This phenomenon is attributed to the lower RANKL/OPG ratio present in the gingival crevicular fluid (GCF) of adult patients, as determined by the enzyme-linked immunosorbent assay (ELISA) method. Furthermore, a correlation was identified among RANK, OPG, and root resorption during orthodontic tooth movement. Notably, patients exhibiting root resorption produced a substantial amount of RANKL at the compressed site[3611].

Among the cytokines implicated in the facilitation of tooth movement is RANKL, a membrane-bound protein located on osteoblasts that binds to RANK on osteoclasts[91], thereby inducing osteoclastogenesis[92]. Conversely, osteoprotegerin (OPG) competes with RANKL for binding to osteoclasts, thereby inhibiting osteoclastogenesis. The process of bone remodeling is thus a balance between the RANKL-RANK system and the OPG compound [12].

PROSTAGLANDIN EFFECT ON TOOTH MOVEMENT

Prostaglandins (PGs) are inflammatory mediators and a paracrine hormone that act on nearby cells; they stimulate bone resorption by directly increasing the number of osteoclasts. In vivo and in vitro experiments were conducted to show clearly the relation between PGs, applied forces, and the acceleration of tooth movement. Yamasaki [94,95] was among the first to investigate the effect of local administration of prostaglandin on rats[94] and monkeys[95] . In addition, experiments done have shown that injections of exogenous PGE2 over an extended period of time caused acceleration of tooth movements in rats[96]. Furthermore, the acceleration rate was not affected by single or multiple injections or between different concentrations of the injected PGE2. However, root resorption was very clearly related to the different concentrations and number of injections given. It has also been shown that the administration of PGE2 in the presence of calcium stabilizes root resorption while accelerating tooth movement [19]. Furthermore, chemically produced PGE2 has been studied in human trials with split-mouth experiments in the first premolar extraction cases. In these experiments the rate of distal retraction of canines was 1.6-fold faster than the control side[19].

Local administration of prostaglandin E1 (PGE1) or prostaglandin E2 (PGE2) in humans, monkeys, and rats has been documented to expedite orthodontic tooth movement. A significant drawback of this method is the pain experienced at the injection site, which has been shown to be mitigated by dissolving prostaglandins in dental lidocaine[18] . Lower concentrations of PGE2, specifically at 0.1 or 1.0 µg, have been demonstrated to effectively enhance orthodontic tooth movement, in contrast to higher concentrations of 5.0, 10.0, or even up to 15 µg, as observed in previous studies. A single injection of PGE2 proved to be as effective in promoting orthodontic tooth movement as multiple injections administered at 2- and 4-week intervals in rats. However, it is noteworthy that higher concentrations of PGE2 were associated with an increased incidence of root resorption [96].

EFFECT OF VITAMIN D3 ON TOOTH MOVEMENT

Vitamin D3 (1,25-dihydroxycholecalciferol) is a significant factor influencing the rate of bone remodeling, and consequently, its impact on the rate of tooth movement has been investigated. Vitamin D3 modulates calcium and phosphate serum levels by enhancing their intestinal absorption and renal reabsorption. Additionally, it facilitates bone deposition and suppresses parathyroid hormone (PTH) release. Based on these mechanisms, it would be anticipated that vitamin D3 would reduce the rate of tooth movement. Contrary to this expectation, research has demonstrated that vitamin D3 can increase the rate of tooth movement when administered locally [14,97] . This effect may be attributed to vitamin

D3's role in augmenting the expression of receptor activator of nuclear factor kappa-B ligand (RANKL) by local cells, thereby activating osteoclasts [98]. A separate group of researchers conducted an experiment in which they administered a vitamin D metabolite to the periodontal ligament (PDL) of cats over several weeks[14]. The findings indicated that vitamin D accelerated tooth movement by 60% compared to the control group. This effect was attributed to an increase in osteoclasts at the pressure site, as observed through histological analysis.

Both 1,25 dihydroxycholecalciferol (1,25-DHCC) and prostaglandin E2 (PGE2) significantly facilitated orthodontic tooth movement in rats, exhibiting distinct differences in their bone remodeling mechanisms. Notably, the researchers determined that 1,25-DHCC was more effective[20] in modulating bone turnover due to its balanced impact on bone formation and resorption. The evidence supporting this conclusion is moderately robust, derived from a controlled experimental design with multiple treatment groups and precise histological measurements, although it is constrained by the small sample size of rats.

RELAXIN EFFECT ON TOOTH MOVEMENT

The effects of relaxin have been the subject of investigation. Relaxin is a hormone that facilitates childbirth by widening the pubic ligaments in females and is hypothesized to be present in cranial sutures and the periodontal ligament (PDL). Its role is primarily associated with the remodeling of soft tissue rather than bone[99]. It has been demonstrated that relaxin increases collagen at tension sites and decreases it at compression sites during orthodontic movement. The remodeling of the PDL by relaxin may potentially reduce the rate of relapse following orthodontic treatment, as suggested by previous studies. Relaxin has been used in rats to increase the rate of tooth movement. Relaxin is capable of reducing the organization level of connective tissues, facilitating rapid separation between adjoining bones. Human relaxin has complex and somewhat contradictory effects on orthodontic tooth movement in rats, primarily altering periodontal ligament (PDL) structure without consistently accelerating tooth movement. Unfortunately, no significant increase in the rate of tooth movement was observed in these studies[100]. Recently, randomized clinical trials involving human subjects were conducted, administering weekly injections of 50 µg of relaxin or a placebo control over an 8-week period.

Tooth movement was assessed weekly using polyvinyl siloxane impressions, which were digitally scanned. The results indicated no significant difference between the relaxin and placebo control groups in terms of acceleration and relapse. However, the precise mechanism by which relaxin accelerates tooth movement remains incompletely understood[45].

EFFECT OF INTERLEUKIN-1 ALPHA AND TUMOR NECROSIS FACTOR

Orthodontic tooth movement (OTM) results from the systematic remodeling of periodontal tissues following the application of mechanical forces. At the cellular level, this remodeling involves bone resorption adjacent to the periodontal ligament (PDL) in the compression zone, bone apposition in the tension zone, and the degeneration and re-establishment of the PDL. Several factors have been identified as contributors to the complex orchestration of tissue remodeling during orthodontic tooth movement. It has been suggested that chemical mediators, such as cytokines, play a significant role. Cytokines are small protein molecules that regulate cell communication and function, actively secreted by various cell types in response to external stimuli. During OTM, these signaling molecules are proposed to be produced by inflammatory cells that migrate from dilated PDL capillaries following the application of orthodontic force. Interleukin (IL)-1 and tumor necrosis factor-alpha (TNF-α) are key mediators in acute-phase inflammatory reactions with overlapping activities. These two pro-inflammatory cytokines are members of the formerly known osteoclast-activating factor (OAF) and have been implicated in the bone remodeling process. IL-1 exists in two isoforms with species differences in osteoclastic activity. In humans, IL-1β constitutes most of the OAF activity, whereas in rodents, IL-1α appears to predominate. Additionally, both isoforms of IL-1 are more potent in stimulating bone resorption than the TNFs.

Tumor necrosis factor-alpha (TNF-α) induces the production of interleukin-1 (IL-1), which in turn stimulates its own synthesis through a positive feedback mechanism. At sites of inflammation, both IL-1 and TNF-α are expressed in significant quantities by macrophages, as well as by various other cell types, including fibroblasts, osteoblasts, and osteoclasts.

These cytokines have been implicated in several chronic inflammatory diseases, such as rheumatoid arthritis, osteomyelitis, and marginal and apical periodontitis, where bone resorption is a primary pathogenetic feature. Moreover, IL-1α and its receptor have been identified as important factors in tissue homeostasis and during physiological tooth movement. Immunohistochemical studies have demonstrated the presence of IL-1α and IL-1β in the periodontal ligament (PDL) of cat canines during the early stages of orthodontic tooth movement, specifically at 12 and 24 hours. In rats, the induction of IL-1β was observed to peak three days following the application of mechanical force. Elevated levels of IL-1 and TNF-α have been detected in the gingival crevicular fluid (GCF) of orthodontic patients, suggesting that these increased cytokine levels reflect the biological responses induced by mechanical stress. The synthesis of IL-1β and TNF-α in GCF during tooth mobilization appeared to stabilize 24 hours after force application, indicating a central role for these cytokines in the initial phase of orthodontic tooth movement. Although substantial data exist on cytokine production during orthodontic tooth movement, there is limited information regarding the specific time frame of cytokine expression. Therefore, the objective of this study was to investigate the expression of IL-1α and TNF-α in dental tissues at 3 hours, 1 day, and 3 days post-orthodontic force application, to provide further insights into the involvement and interaction of these cytokines in the early stages of orthodontic tooth movement[13].

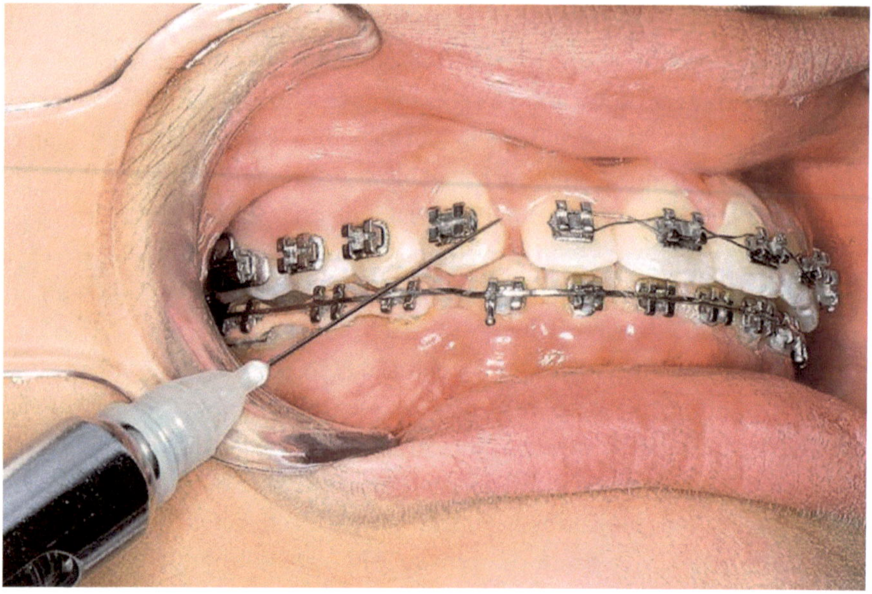

FIG 2: Injection of a biomodulator in the periodontium

LIMITATIONS

The utilization of chemical agents to accelerate tooth movement presents several challenges. Foremost, these agents elicit systemic effects, raising substantial concerns regarding their safety in clinical applications. Furthermore, the majority of these agents possess a limited half-life, necessitating repeated applications, a practice deemed impractical in orthodontic clinics. Additionally, achieving a uniform distribution of the agent across the alveolar bone surface at the compression site remains a significant challenge. Inconsistent distribution can alter the resorption pattern and, consequently, impact the biomechanics of tooth movement[101].

CHAPTER V

PHYSICAL STIMULATION

MECHANICAL STIMULATION

A method that has been suggested to accelerate tooth movement involves the use of high-frequency, low-magnitude forces, commonly referred to as vibration, applied to teeth undergoing orthodontic treatment. The hypothesis is predicated on the assumption that orthodontic forces directly target bone, implying that enhancing mechanical stimulation could potentially expedite tooth movement. However, while this approach may be effective under specific conditions, the foundational assumptions of this technique are flawed. As previously discussed, the belief that tooth movement is a direct result of bone cells responding to mechanical stimulation is incorrect. Therefore, optimizing mechanical stimulation based on the activity of bone cells, particularly osteocytes, is not a valid strategy. According to this biological principle, the application of vibration and orthodontic forces will not facilitate the movement of an ankylosed tooth. Moreover, research on long bone and alveolar bone[102] demonstrates that vibration induces osteogenic effects, increasing bone density without any resorptive effect, which should logically impede rather than hasten tooth movement. Although there is limited evidence supporting the influence of vibration on the rate of tooth movement [32], it is plausible that high-frequency, low-magnitude forces during orthodontic treatment may activate a pathway distinct from its direct impact on bone. If this is the case, the frequency dependence of the stimulant is questionable, and existing literature should not be used to justify the application of vibration during tooth movement.

HEAT, LIGHT, ELECTRIC CURRENTS, AND MAGNETIC FIELDS AND LASER

Initial research on the use of heat and light in orthodontic tooth movement[103] has shown a potential increase in the speed of tooth movement. Similarly, animals subjected to prolonged light exposure also demonstrate a heightened rate of tooth movement[104]. Nevertheless, the degree of this acceleration was either negligible or could be more accurately attributed to systemic effects rather than localized influences. The application of small electric currents has been proposed as a method to enhance tooth movement rates. While some studies have found no significant changes in tooth movement[105], others have reported notable increases[106]. Similarly, investigations into static magnetic fields have produced mixed outcomes, with some studies reporting an increase in tooth movement[107] and others finding no effect[108]. According to the piezoelectric theory, some researchers recommend the use of pulsed electromagnetic fields to accelerate tooth movement[109]. Indeed, animals exposed to this form of stimulation during orthodontic procedures exhibit increased tooth movement[110]. However, the precise mechanism responsible for this effect remains unclear, and the roles of inflammation and osteoclast activation have not been thoroughly investigated.

CHAPTER VI

DEVICE-ASSISTED APPROACH

An alternative strategy to hasten tooth movement is the implementation of device-assisted therapy. Although surgical techniques vary, they invariably involve some level of invasiveness and are thus linked to potential complications. As a result, non-invasive methods have become increasingly prominent. These methods include the application of direct electric currents, pulsed electromagnetic fields, static magnetic fields, resonance vibration, and low-level laser therapy, with the latter being the most extensively researched and showing the most promising results. The foundation for using physical methods is based on the bone bending theory, which posits that orthodontic forces cause bone bending and generate bioelectrical potentials. Zengo's research on canine alveolar bone revealed that the concave side becomes negatively charged, attracting osteoblasts, while the convex side becomes positively charged, attracting osteoclasts. This bioelectrical potential is produced when discontinuous forces are applied, prompting the investigation of cyclic forces and vibrations.

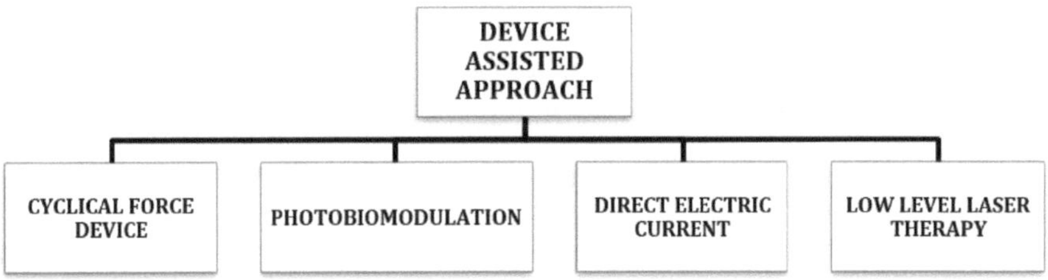

CYCLICAL FORCE DEVICE EFFECT ON TOOTH MOVEMENT

Kau et al[43]. conducted a study utilizing a cyclical force device with patients, achieving a tooth movement rate of 2 to 3 mm per month. This device functioned at a vibration frequency of 20 to 30 Hz and was applied for 20 minutes daily, employing soft pulse technology[49]. The process of orthodontic tooth movement involves bone resorption on the compressed side of the periodontal ligament (PDL) and bone formation on the stretched side, induced by therapeutic mechanical stress. Orthodontic treatments are often lengthy, leading to challenges such as caries, periodontal disease, and extended treatment durations, which can be burdensome for patients. Moreover, there is a strong correlation between the total treatment duration and root resorption. Therefore, accelerating alveolar bone remodeling during orthodontic treatment is essential to reduce the therapy duration. Various strategies have been explored to expedite tooth movement, including physical methods like low-energy laser irradiation and magnetic fields, as well as pharmacological methods involving prostaglandin E2 (PGE2)5-7 and 1,25-$(OH)_2D_3$ injections. However, these approaches have been associated with side effects such as local pain, severe root resorption, and drug-induced adverse effects. The initial cellular response to mechanical stress in vitro occurs within 30 minutes. We have aimed to trigger these initial cellular responses by applying resonance vibrational stimulation to a tooth and its periodontal tissue. Additionally, resonance vibration that aligns with the natural frequency of the first molar and its periodontal tissue enhances the stimulation of the periodontal tissue. Consequently, we hypothesized that applying resonance vibration during orthodontic tooth movement could accelerate tooth movement by enhancing cellular activity in the PDL. Our study aimed to examine the effects of resonance vibration stimulation on the rate of tooth movement and root resorption during experimental tooth movement in rats, and to elucidate the cellular and molecular mechanisms that facilitate the acceleration of tooth movement.

A new product, Acceledent, has recently been launched in the market, employing advanced technology. This device includes an activator, which is the primary component responsible for delivering vibration impulses. It is equipped with a USB interface, enabling connection to a computer for monitoring patient usage, and features a mouthpiece that makes contact with the teeth. The device is portable and can be charged similarly to other electronic devices, requiring a daily usage of 20 minutes. Several case studies have indicated that the use of this device can reduce treatment durations by 30-40%[49].

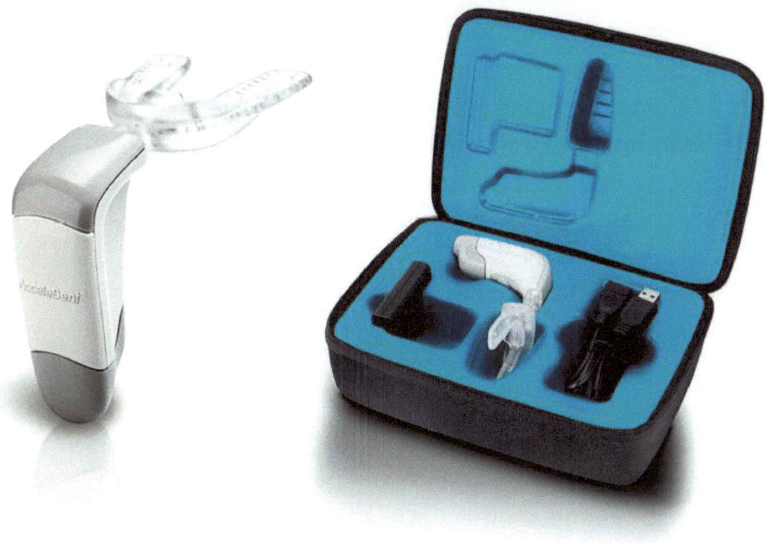

FIG 3: Acceledent device along with its USB interface which is used to connect it to a computer

PHOTOBIOMODULATION

Light-accelerated orthodontics (LAO) is a method situated within the realm of photobiomodulation, also referred to as low-level light therapy. The terms photobiomodulation and LAO are often used interchangeably to denote the specific wavelength range, intensity, and light penetration, thereby distinguishing them from other light-based dental treatment techniques. LAO shows potential for noninvasive stimulation of the dentoalveolar complex, with a possible effect on the production of adenosine triphosphate (ATP) by mitochondrial cells. The hypothesis is that an increase in ATP at a localized site will trigger cells to engage in a remodeling process due to heightened metabolic activity. Cytochrome oxidase e, which mediates ATP production, is upregulated twofold by infrared light. During the phase of tooth movement, the increased availability of ATP supports more efficient cell turnover, resulting in enhanced remodeling and expedited tooth movement.

Additionally, LAO may operate through augmented vascular activity, which contributes to rapid bone turnover and is responsive to light. Several clinical case series have indicated that LAO enhances the speed of canine movement, alleviates pain, and significantly accelerates the retraction of treated canines. Nonetheless, some studies have raised questions regarding its efficacy[49].

The Extra-oral Ortho Pulse LED, developed by Biolux Research in Vancouver, Canada, is an external device designed to emit near-infrared light at a continuous wavelength of 850 nm. The device irradiates the cheek surface with a power density of 60 mW/cm² for durations of either 20 or 30 minutes per day, or alternatively, 60 minutes per week, to achieve total energy densities of 72, 108, or 216 J/cm², respectively. The light is generated using industry-standard light-emitting diodes (LEDs), which are configured in arrays to effectively cover the target area of the alveolus in both the maxilla and mandible.

The device comprises three primary components:

1) A compact handheld controller that contains the microprocessor, menu-driven software, and an LCD screen. This controller is programmable by the investigator to set the number of treatment sessions and their duration. The user interface informs the patient of the number of sessions completed and the remaining time in each session. The controller connects to the power mains via a medically approved, UL-certified power supply.

2) A set of four extra-oral treatment arrays, each equipped with a flexible printed circuit board and a series of LEDs mounted on a contoured heat sink and an infrared-transmissible plastic lens, with conductive cables linking to the controller.

3) A headset resembling an eyeglass support structure, designed to be worn by the patient on a daily or weekly basis, featuring attachment and adjustment mechanisms to position the treatment arrays appropriately for the individual patient.

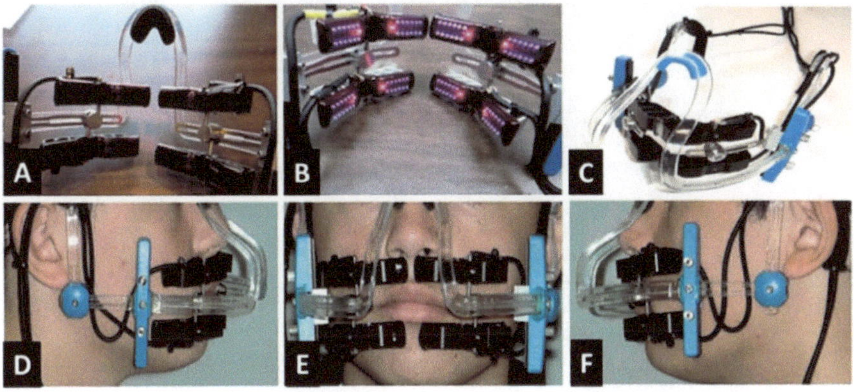

FIG 4: Device components and a clinical presentation. (A, B) A set of four extra-oral treatment arrays, each with a flexible printed circuit board and a set of LEDs mounted on a contoured heat sink and infrared-transmissible plastic lens, with conductive cables to the controller. (C) A headset similar to an eyeglass support structure to be worn by the patient on a daily or weekly basis, with attachment and adjustment mechanisms to position the treatment arrays in the appropriate location for the given patient. (D, E, F) Clinical presentation of the device[49]

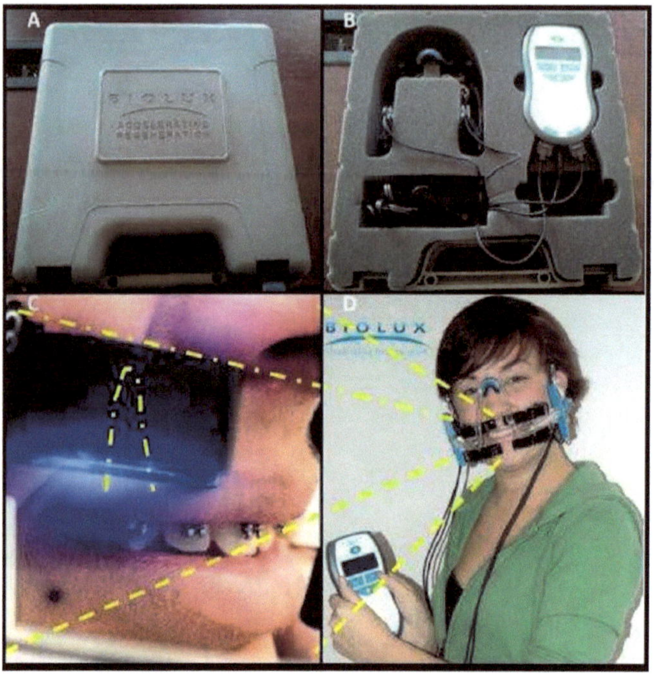

FIG 5: Biolux Machine[111]

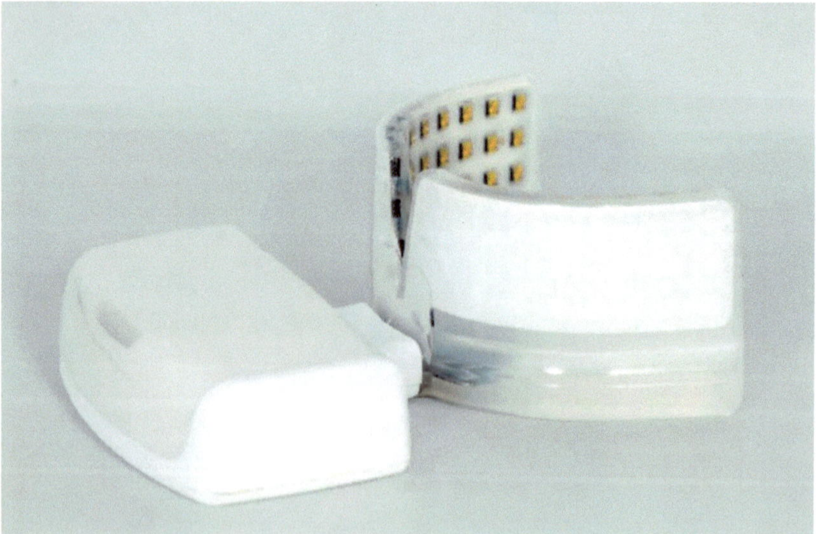

FIG 6: New Biolux OrthoPulse™ LED device

The LED device is described as follows: A) The device is encased in a hard plastic shell with sponge insulation, which is provided to each patient to mitigate impact damage. B) Each device comprises a face mask equipped with LED arrays, a power supply, and a handheld controller unit. C) The face mask is designed to ensure a secure and consistent positioning on the face, with the LED arrays aligned parallel to the patient's occlusal plane. The LED array is strategically positioned and programmed to target the root of the tooth undergoing retraction, as well as the extraction space into which the tooth is being moved, on only one side of the face. D) Although the LED illumination is visibly noticeable in C, it is not visible to the naked eye.

The device administers all light treatments extraorally. Any heat produced as a by-product of light generation is monitored and maintained below the thresholds established by electro-medical device safety standards. The device ensures patient compliance by activating the treatment arrays only when worn by the patient, allowing the physician to access compliance data during each patient visit. The processor records the duration of device activation in minutes and logs the number of sessions the patient utilizes the device. The application of light and continuous forces to the dentoalveolar complex facilitates optimal alignment rates. Photobiomodulation enhances the rate of tooth movement, achieving a rate of 1.12 mm per week[49].

Carlos Goulart and colleagues conducted a double-blind study to assess the impact of gallium-aluminum-arsenide (GaAlAs) laser irradiation on the rate of orthodontic movement in canine premolars[25]. The study involved eighteen dogs, which were divided into two groups following the extraction of their third molars. An orthodontic device was installed between the first molar and the second premolar to ensure stabilization. In Group I, the right side was subjected to laser irradiation at a dosage of 5.25 J/cm², while the left side served as the control. Group II underwent a similar procedure, but with a higher irradiation dosage of 35.0 J/cm². The laser treatments were administered every 7 days, culminating in a total of nine sessions. Measurements of the orthodontic space were taken every 21 days. The findings indicated that the 5.25 J/cm² dosage significantly accelerated orthodontic movement during the initial observation period, spanning 0 to 21 days ($p<0.05$). Conversely, the 35.0 J/cm² dosage was found to impede orthodontic movement in the treated group compared to the control group during both the first and second observation periods, from 0 to 42 days ($p<0.05$). The researchers concluded that photoradiation at a dosage of 5.25 J/cm² may enhance orthodontic movement, whereas a higher dosage of 35.0 J/cm² may have a retarding effect[25].

DIRECT ELECTRIC CURRENT EFFECT ON TOOTH MOVEMENT

Kim et al. conducted a study demonstrating that electrical current can expedite orthodontic tooth movement. In their experiment, an electrical device was installed in the maxilla to administer a direct current of 20 microns. The maxillary canine on one side was designated as the experimental subject, while the canine on the opposite side served as the control. The experimental canine was exposed to both orthodontic force and electrical current, whereas the control canine was subjected only to orthodontic force. The electrical current was applied to the experimental canines for 5 hours each day. After one month, the authors observed that the cumulative movement of the experimental group was significantly greater, measuring 2.42 ± 0.26 mm, compared to 1.89 ± 0.27 mm in the control group. The electrical current was delivered to the mucosa of the canines through a fixed electrical appliance assembly, operating at 20 MA for 5 hours daily[112].

Piezoelectric currents, which arise in mechanically stressed bone, have been associated with the activation of bone cells. In light of this, Davidovitch et al[106]. conducted a study to assess the potential of exogenous electric currents in enhancing the rate of orthodontic tooth movement and to investigate their effect on periodontal cyclic nucleotides. In their experiment, maxillary canines in five cats were subjected to an 80 g force. Two separate groups, each comprising five cats, received an electric-orthodontic treatment on one maxillary canine for periods of 7 and 14 days, respectively.

The findings revealed that teeth exposed to both mechanical force and electric currents moved at a significantly faster rate than those subjected to force alone. Notably, increased bone resorption was observed near the anode, corresponding to the periodontal ligament compression site, while bone formation was more evident near the cathode, corresponding to the periodontal ligament tension site. Furthermore, the addition of electric stimulation to mechanical force resulted in heightened staining for cyclic nucleotides. The study concludes that the application of localized electric currents may effectively accelerate orthodontic tooth movement[106,113].

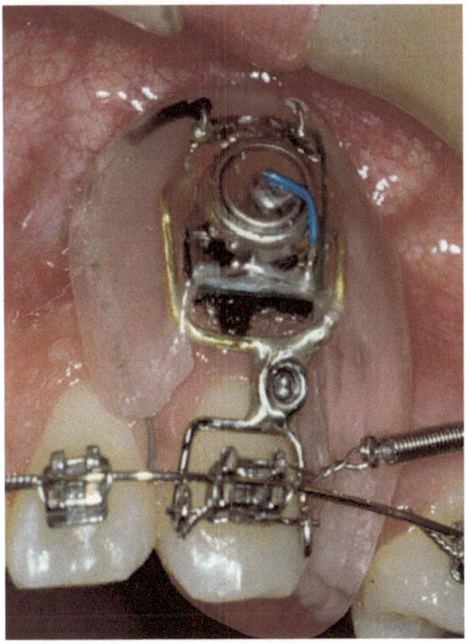

FIG 7: Fixed type electric appliance set up on the upper left canine[33]

LOW-LEVEL LASER THERAPY

Recent academic discourse has increasingly examined the influence of low-level laser therapy (LLLT) on the acceleration of tooth movement. LLLT is a therapeutic modality that utilizes low-level lasers or light-emitting diodes to influence cellular processes. Within the realm of conventional medicine, LLLT remains a subject of debate, with ongoing investigations seeking to establish its efficacy. Furthermore, there is ongoing discussion regarding the optimal parameters for LLLT, including dose, wavelength, timing, pulsing, and duration[114]. The therapeutic effects of LLLT are believed to be restricted to certain wavelengths[115], and its administration below a specific dose threshold appears to lack effectiveness[116].

The underlying mechanisms of LLLT are not fully elucidated and may occasionally conflict with the requirements for orthodontic tooth movement. For example, LLLT has the potential to mitigate pain associated with inflammation by dose-dependently reducing levels of PGE2, IL-1, and TNF-α, thereby diminishing the influx of inflammatory cells such as neutrophils, as well as oxidative stress and edema[117]. Given the anti-inflammatory and osteogenic characteristics of LLLT[118], its use to expedite tooth movement is contentious. Some studies have reported enhanced rates of tooth movement[44], while others have found no significant effect[119].

The anti-inflammatory properties of LLLT might delay tooth movement, whereas its proliferative effects could potentially increase osteoblast numbers. Conversely, certain studies have observed an increase in osteoclast numbers during LLLT application in conjunction with orthodontic tooth movement[120], a finding that cannot be attributed to a proliferative effect of lasers, as osteoclasts derive from precursor cells rather than the proliferation of mature osteoclasts, as some have proposed.

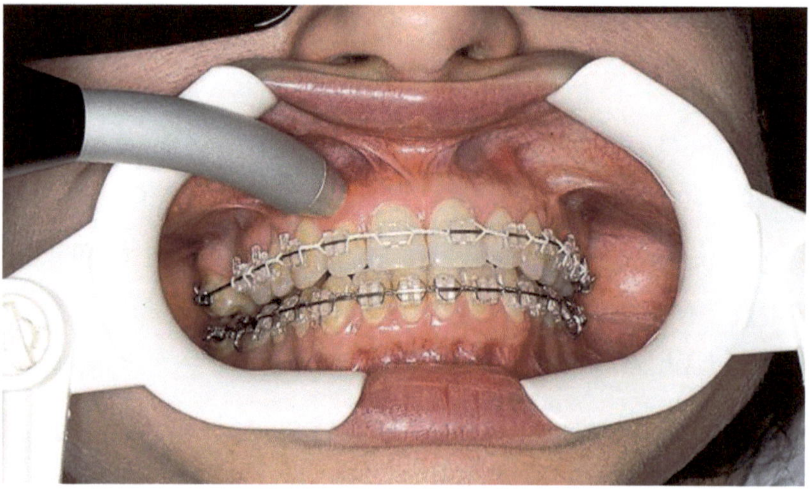

FIG 8: Low-level laser therapy[121]

Research involving animal models has indicated that low-level laser therapy (LLLT) can facilitate the acceleration of tooth movement. Clinical trials have also been conducted with varying laser intensities, resulting in a range of outcomes. LLLT is considered a promising technique for enhancing tooth movement, as it promotes bone remodeling without causing harm to the periodontium. Specifically, a laser wavelength of 800 nm and an output power of 0.25 mW have been shown to significantly stimulate bone metabolism, promote rapid ossification, and increase tooth movement by 1.5 times in rat studies. In a recent clinical trial, the use of a continuous wave mode laser at 800 nm, with an output of 0.25 mW and a 10-second exposure, resulted in a 1.3-fold increase in tooth movement compared to the control group[44]. Another study by Kau et al[49]. involving 90 participants (73 test subjects and 17 controls) reported a weekly change of 1.12 mm in the test group, compared to 0.49 mm in the control group. Despite these findings, there remains a lack of consensus regarding LLLT, necessitating further research to establish the optimal energy, wavelength, and duration for its effective application.

Cruz et al[22] were the pioneers in conducting a human study to investigate the impact of low-intensity laser therapy on orthodontic tooth movement. Their findings indicated that the irradiated canines were retracted at a rate 34% greater than the control canines over a period of 60 days. In 2013, Gauri Doshi Mehta et al[44]. employed a split-mouth design, utilizing an 800 nm laser for 10 seconds on the canine, both buccally and lingually, which required distalization following the extraction of the first premolar. A Ni-Ti closed coil spring was used to deliver a constant force of 150 g from the first molar tube hook to the power arm of the canine bracket, secured with a ligature tie to the bracket.

The laser employed was a semiconductor (aluminium gallium arsenide) diode (model LA3D0001.1; LAMBDA S.p.A., Vicenza, Italy) emitting infrared radiation with a wavelength of 808±10 nm, operated in accordance with the manufacturer's recommendations. The study also aimed to explore the analgesic properties of laser therapy. For analgesic purposes, the settings were adjusted to a wavelength of 800 nm, a continuous wave mode, an output power of 0.7 mW, and an exposure time of 30 seconds. For bio-stimulation, the parameters were set at a wavelength of 800 nm, a continuous wave mode, an output power of 0.25 mW, and an exposure time of 10 seconds. The total energy density (dose) at each application was 8 J (2 × 40 s × 100 mW). After 6 months, peri-apical radiographs of the laser-treated (experimental) and control side canines revealed no undesirable changes in the adjacent periodontal ligaments and alveolar bones. Vitality tests of the retracted canines were also positive. Three models were created for each patient. On these models, the mesial cusp tips of the first molar and the canine served as reference points. The distance between the first molar and the canine was measured on all three models for each patient using a digital caliper accurate to 0.02 mm. These distances were recorded at T0 (after completion of alignment and leveling: day 1 of canine retraction), T1 (at the end of 3 months of canine retraction), and T2 (upon completion of canine retraction on the experimental side).

The study demonstrated a highly significant positive difference in the rates of tooth movement on the experimental side compared to the control side. At three months, the mean increase in the rates of tooth movement was 54% in the maxillary arch and 58% in the mandibular arch. Following canine retraction, the mean increase in the rate of tooth movement was 29% in the maxillary arch and 31% in the mandibular arch. A significant reduction in pain scores was recorded using a Visual Analogue Scale. The study employed a semiconductor with a wavelength of 800 nm, continuous wave mode, an output power of 0.25 mW, and an exposure time of 10 seconds.

This choice was informed by the findings of Takeda and Bradley et al., which indicated significant bio-stimulatory effects on bone metabolism at this dosage, whereas higher dosages exhibited bio-inhibitory effects, and lower dosages yielded non-significant results. Conversely, Limpanichkul et al. (2006) reported that low-level laser therapy had no additive effect on orthodontic tooth movement, potentially due to the higher energy density of 25 J per square centimeter used in their study. Various studies on low-level laser therapy have reported increases in orthodontic tooth movement ranging from 30% to 60%. The discrepancies among these studies appear to stem from variations in the frequency of laser application, laser intensity, and the method of force application on the tooth. In this study, a Ga-Al-As diode laser (Osada Inc., Tokyo, Japan) with a wavelength of 810 nm and continuous waves at 100 mW output power was utilized. These irradiation conditions were determined by previous experiments (Kawasaki and Shimizu, 2000). The laser beam was delivered via a 0.6 mm diameter optical fiber, and irradiation was administered under anesthesia by placing the optical fiber tip in contact with the mesial, buccal, and palatal sides of the gingiva in the area of the upper right first molar undergoing orthodontic tooth movement. Irradiation was performed for 3 minutes at each point (a total of 9 minutes) once a day on days 0–7 (a total of eight times). The total energy corresponding to an exposure time of 9 minutes was 54.0 J[122].

S. Na et al[123] found that different cell types respond uniquely to varying light doses, with low doses (1 J/cm²) potentially enhancing cellular activities, while higher doses can inhibit cell viability. Similarly, C. Cotomacio et al[124] observed that lower energy protocols sometimes produced better healing outcomes compared to higher energy treatments. These studies underscore the complexity of radiation dosing and the importance of precise energy delivery in therapeutic applications.

The application of low-level laser therapy is regarded as an effective adjunct in orthodontic treatment, as it significantly accelerates the rate of tooth movement and substantially reduces the level of pain experienced[26].

CHAPTER VII

SURGICAL APPROACH

In 1931, Bichmalyr proposed a surgical method that incorporated orthodontic devices to swiftly address severe maxillary protrusion. This approach initially involved the removal of bone wedges to create space for the retraction of the roots of the maxillary anterior teeth. In 1959, Köle expanded upon this method by integrating additional movements, such as crossbite correction and space closure. He asserted that it was possible to manipulate bony segments by utilizing the crowns of teeth as levers, as these segments were linked only by less-dense medullary bone.

The surgical approach represents a clinically effective technique for adult patients, particularly when the duration of orthodontic treatment is a critical consideration for specific patient groups. The periodontal ligament (PDL) and alveolar bone remodeling are essential parameters in tooth movement, with bone turnover known to increase following bone grafting, fracture, and osteotomy.

Orthodontic forces trigger an aseptic inflammatory response[28,125], during which a variety of cytokines and chemokines are activated, significantly contributing to osteoclastogenesis. It is plausible to propose that augmenting the activity of these factors could markedly enhance the rate of tooth movement. Inducing trauma in the area of tooth movement is one method to stimulate a heightened release of cytokines and chemokines. The literature describes various approaches that induce different levels of trauma, which have been demonstrated to affect the rate of tooth movement. The effectiveness of these interventions is linked to the role of inflammation and osteoclastogenesis in facilitating tooth movement. While these methods activate similar biological pathways, they vary in the degree of tissue trauma and invasiveness, leading to different levels of complications, pain, and discomfort. Crucially, not all these procedures are straightforward to execute or easily repeatable, which can limit the orthodontist's ability to integrate their accelerating effects into the biomechanical design and anchorage requirements of each patient's treatment plan.

Various surgical methods have been investigated to accelerate tooth movement, including interseptal alveolar surgery, osteotomy, corticotomy, micro osteoperforation and the piezocision technique[126].

INTERSEPTAL ALVEOLAR SURGERY

Interseptal alveolar surgery, commonly referred to as distraction osteogenesis, encompasses two primary techniques: the distraction of the periodontal ligament (PDL) and the distraction of the dentoalveolar bone. Rapid canine distraction exemplifies both methods. The foundational principles of distraction osteogenesis were initially derived from early research on limb lengthening. This approach was later adapted from surgical interventions for craniofacial skeletal dysplasia to promote accelerated tooth movement.

Distraction osteogenesis is a technique that involves the manipulation of a healing bone by extending an osteotomized region before calcification occurs. This process encourages the formation of additional bone and surrounding soft tissue, which is beneficial for correcting facial deformities. The method presents two primary advantages: (1) it allows for greater movement distances than traditional orthognathic surgery, and (2) it enables the enlargement of underdeveloped jaws at a younger age. However, a significant drawback is the lack of precision in movement. While distraction facilitates the forward movement of the mandible or maxilla, it does not allow for the precise positioning of the jaw or teeth, a capability that is standard in orthognathic procedures[127].

a
b
c
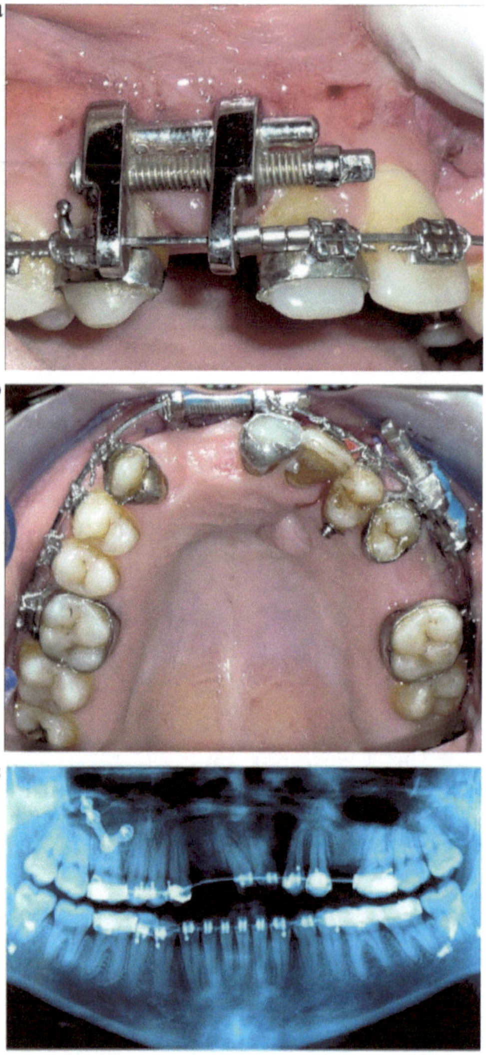

FIG 9: (a)Distractor in the mouth. (b) Occlusal view showing the undisturbed arch form at the end of distraction. (c) New bone formation at the distraction sites[128]

Interseptal alveolar surgery, or distraction osteogenesis, can be classified into periodontal ligament (PDL) distraction or dentoalveolar bone distraction, with rapid canine distraction exemplifying both. The concept of distraction osteogenesis originated from early limb lengthening studies and was later adapted for surgical interventions in craniofacial skeletal dysplasia, particularly concerning rapid tooth movement.

In the procedure of rapid canine distraction involving the periodontal ligament (PDL), the interseptal bone located distal to the canine is surgically undermined simultaneously with the extraction of the first premolars. This approach is designed to decrease resistance at the pressure site. The method involves substituting compact bone with woven bone, thereby facilitating more efficient and expedited tooth movement due to the reduced resistance of the bone[39]. Observations indicate that these rapid movements are most prominent during the initial stages of tooth movement, particularly within the first week. In this technique, the interseptal bone is undermined to a thickness of 1 to 1.5 mm distal to the canine following the extraction of the first premolar, and the socket is deepened using a round bur to correspond with the length of the canine. The retraction of the canine is accomplished through the activation of an intraoral device immediately following surgery.

It has been documented that complete retraction of the canine, measuring 6 to 7 mm, is achieved within three weeks into the socket of the extracted first premolars[39]. The principle of rapid canine distraction of the dentoalveolar bone is analogous to that of PDL distraction, with additional dissection and osteotomies conducted at the vestibule. Across various studies, both techniques have been demonstrated to accelerate tooth movement without significant evidence of root resorption, ankylosis, or root fracture. However, there are discrepancies in the results concerning the electrical vitality test of the retracted canines. Liou[13] reported that 9 out of 26 teeth exhibited positive vitality, whereas Sukurica[129] reported that 7 out of 20 showed positive vitality after six months of retraction. The current evidence indicates the method is generally safe, but pulpal response remains an area of ongoing investigation.

PIEZOCISION

Given the invasive nature of the corticotomy procedure, Dibart et al[139]. introduced a novel, minimally invasive technique known as piezocision. This method involves microincisions restricted to the buccal side, facilitating the use of a piezoelectric knife and selective tunneling, which permits both hard and soft tissue grafting. Typically, piezocision is performed one week following the placement of orthodontic appliances.

The procedure entails making vertical incisions buccally and interproximally. The central portion of the incision, located between the roots, allows for the insertion of the piezoelectric knife. Subsequently, a piezotome is introduced into the gingival openings, enabling a piezoelectrical corticotomy of 3 mm. Hard or soft tissue grafts can then be incorporated through a tunneling procedure. In regions necessitating bone augmentation, a tunneling technique is employed using an elevator inserted between the incisions to create adequate space for the placement of graft material. Depending on the number and location of the piezoincisions, this procedure may result in significant trauma and subsequent inflammation. However, suturing is generally not required, except in areas where stabilization of the graft material is necessary. The patient is prescribed an antibiotic and mouthwash regimen.

Piezocision serves as an adjunctive technique for addressing various malocclusions and facilitating expedited orthodontic treatment in adults. Due to its minimally invasive nature compared to corticotomy, it enjoys a high level of patient acceptance, requires a shorter surgical duration, and results in reduced postoperative discomfort. In 2013, Dibart and colleagues[139] demonstrated an increased rate of tooth movement in their animal study, and preliminary human studies are currently underway to establish correlations with the animal findings.

Similar to corticotomy, this procedure necessitates the involvement of a specialist other than the orthodontist, such as a periodontist or oral surgeon, which incurs additional costs for the patient. This factor serves as a deterrent to the repeated application required for sustained accelerated movement following the subsidence of inflammation. Consequently, piezoincisions are not practical for routine orthodontic practice for both patients and clinicians.

In 2013, Jofre et al[50]. proposed a method known as the Minimally Invasive Rapid Orthodontic (MIRO) procedure to mitigate the risk of root damage. MIRO reduces orthodontic treatment time while minimizing surgical invasiveness[50]. The technique uses microincisions and localized piezoelectric corticotomies, which avoid the extensive tissue disruption of traditional methods. The technique involves the use of metal wires as guides for the placement of incisions and subsequent corticotomies. Metal guides are positioned between each tooth, perpendicular to the main arch wire, and digital radiographs are taken to ensure that the metal guides do not overlap the tooth roots. Upon confirmation, incisions and piezoelectric corticotomy are performed using the pins as guides. The clinical outcomes of MIRO retain the benefits of accelerated orthodontics as described by Chung et al., while being significantly less traumatic due to its flapless nature, thereby reducing both trauma and recovery time.

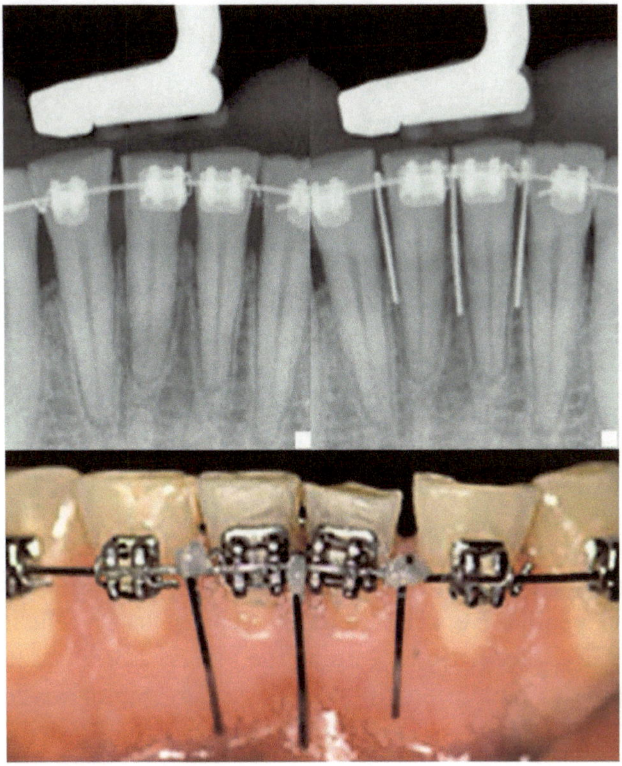

FIG 10: Radiographic metal guides were positioned between each tooth, and digital radiographs were obtained to ensure that the metal pin did not project over the tooth roots[50].

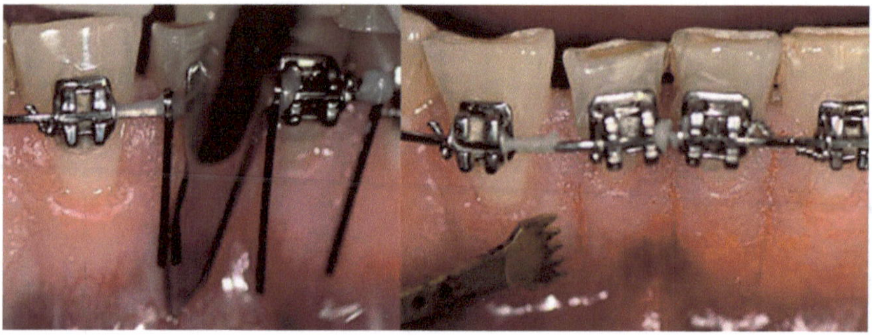

FIG 11: The metal pin allows an accurate mucoperiosteal incision 2 mm below the papilla. Vertical corticotomies were performed using an ultrasonic microsaw OT7.

A systematic review by T. Fu et al.,[140] in 2019 found flapless corticotomy procedures increased tooth movement rates, with mean treatment time reduced by 68.42 days. Additionally, MIRO enhances precision by utilizing radiographic surgical guides, which facilitate accurate corticotomy and prevent damage to vital structures and teeth.

The standardized surgical protocol[141] stipulates that only patients with periodontal health are eligible for the procedure. Prior to the intervention, comprehensive information regarding the potential benefits and risks was provided to each patient, followed by the acquisition of written informed consent. On the day before the surgery, patients were instructed to use a 0.12% chlorhexidine mouthwash twice, once in the morning and once in the evening. Just before the surgery, patients rinsed with 0.12% chlorhexidine for one minute, and the peribuccal region was cleansed with gauze soaked in chlorhexidine. All surgeries were performed under local anesthesia, specifically using lidocaine hydrochloride 2% with epinephrine 1:100,000. Radiographic metal guides were placed between each tooth, and digital radiographs were obtained to confirm that the metal pin did not extend over the tooth roots. This metal pin was utilized as an accurate guide for executing mucoperiosteal incisions, which began 2 mm below the papilla. An ultrasonic microsaw OT7 (Piezosurgery, Mectron Medical Technology) was employed over the incision site. With bone 1 cutting power and an irrigation solution pump set to level 4, vertical corticotomies were conducted following the gingival incision line.

Following the corticotomies, patients were advised to maintain a soft diet and avoid using mouth rinse for 24 hours. No anti-inflammatory medication was prescribed. Follow-up appointments were scheduled for 24 hours post-surgery, on day 7 and then biweekly for a month, with adjustments made as necessary.

CORTICOTOMY

Corticotomy is a surgical technique designed to accelerate orthodontic tooth movement by selectively cutting cortical bone while preserving medullary bone, thereby reducing bone resistance to tooth movement [130]. The procedure induces a regional acceleratory phenomenon that temporarily increases bone tissue turnover. While studies confirm the technique can statistically accelerate tooth movement, the evidence quality remains low due to methodological limitations. Most research suggests tooth movement can be accelerated by approximately one-third of conventional treatment time[131], with acceleration effects typically lasting 2-3 months[132].

The technique of corticotomy is characterized by its invasive and traumatic nature. This method involves exposing the alveolar bone through the reflection of an extensive gingival tissue flap, followed by multiple deep incisions and perforations into the cortical and trabecular bone between the dental roots[133], executed with a rotary high-speed instrument.

This procedure induces a substantial inflammatory response due to the significant bone trauma incurred. Consequently, it is unsurprising that corticotomies have been demonstrated to expedite tooth movement in rat animal models[134]. The anticipated levels of cytokine activation are the highest among techniques of a similar category, which may be advantageous in cases of mild to moderate crowding where only straightforward leveling and aligning mechanics are required. This can be accomplished with light wires when complex mechanics are unnecessary.

W. M. Wilcko et al., 2001[16]. confirmed a transient localized demineralization-remineralization process in corticotomized patients, consistent with the regional acceleratory phenomenon (RAP) Their computed tomographic evaluation revealed that tooth movement involves a dynamic bone remodeling process, where bone undergoes reversible demineralization rather than rigid "block" movement T. Wilcko et al., 2008[135].

Also W. M. Wilcko et al., 2001[16] directly observed that during orthodontic treatment, the bone matrix becomes malleable, with surface and internal demineralization followed by remineralization. This challenges previous assumptions about bone rigidity and provides a nuanced understanding of bone's adaptive capabilities during mechanical stress. The findings are particularly significant in explaining accelerated orthodontic tooth movement mechanisms.

The efficacy of this technique in expediting tooth movement has been substantiated by numerous researchers. Additionally, it facilitates bone augmentation, thereby mitigating the risk of periodontal defects that may occur due to a thin alveolar bone. Although clinical cases have been documented in support of this technique, it is important to note that despite the potentially favorable initial biological response, significant complications are associated with this method[101].

1. The aggressive and invasive characteristics of this procedure render it challenging for patients to accept repeated applications at various stages of treatment.

2. It represents the least cost-effective option for both patients and clinicians.

3. This procedure is time-intensive and necessitates the longest recovery period.

4. Due to its aggressive nature, integrating this procedure at different treatment stages, where the target of movement may vary, is exceedingly difficult. Consequently, it is not advantageous during routine orthodontic treatment, as different teeth require movement at different treatment stages.

5. If not employed judiciously, it can compromise anchorage.

6. The catabolic effect induced by this method is substantial and may exceed the requirements at the stage of its application, resulting in unnecessary trauma to healthy bone and surrounding structures.

7. The subsequent anabolic effect will be as significant as the catabolic effect, promoting bone formation that can interfere with tooth movement during subsequent treatment stages.

Corticision as a minimally invasive technique for accelerating orthodontic tooth movement. Y. Park et al.,[67] in 2016 defines corticision as a "cortical bone incision" procedure performed without flap elevation. C. Charavet et al.,[136] in 2019 confirms it as one of several minimally invasive techniques developed to decrease orthodontic treatment time. Irfan

Qamruddin et al.,[137] in 2015 categorizes it among the "flapless corticision" procedures to enhance tooth movement velocity.This method employed a reinforced scalpel and mallet to penetrate the gingiva and cortical bone. While this technique did induce the Regional Acceleratory Phenomenon (RAP) effect, it presented certain limitations, such as the inability to place grafts, and the malleting procedure was associated with postoperative dizziness[138].

Although this technique reportedly offers postoperative stability and improved retention, further studies are necessary. The primary drawbacks of these surgical techniques are their invasiveness, and the acceleration effect is limited to the initial 3 to 4 months, subsequently declining to levels comparable to the controls.

PERIODONTALLY ACCELERATED OSTEOGENIC ORTHODONTICS

The term "Wilckodontics," also known as periodontally accelerated osteogenic orthodontics (PAOO), refers to a synergistic approach between orthodontic and periodontal disciplines[142]. This method allows for the rapid movement of teeth through bone by aligning with the principles of periodontal regenerative surgery. The benefits of this approach include 1) expedited tooth movement[143] 2) reduced discomfort associated with orthodontic appliances 3) enhanced stability through the development of a novel local osseous phenotype. In this procedure, surgical trauma induces the release of inflammatory mediators, leading to vasodilation of blood vessels and increased recruitment of osteoclasts at the surgical sites. Consequently, this accelerates bone remodeling. Conversely, corticotomy reduces bone mineral density, thereby decreasing the resistance of dentoalveolar tissues to orthodontic forces and increasing the risk of root resorption.

The exploration of surgically assisted orthodontic tooth movement dates back to the 1800s. In 1893, L.C. Bryan pioneered the description of corticotomy-facilitated tooth movement, as recorded in a textbook by S.H. Guiliford[144]. A pivotal development in this domain was introduced by Henrich Kole in 1959. Kole identified that the primary obstacle to tooth movement was the continuity and thickness of the dense cortical bone. This insight led to the "bony block movement" theory, where he proposed that by disrupting the cortical bone's continuity, he was effectively creating and mobilizing bone blocks containing the teeth. His method involved a combination of radicular corticotomy and supra-apical osteotomy, focusing on the cortical bone and including buccal and lingual interproximal vertical corticotomy cuts. These vertical cuts, positioned approximately 1 mm below the root apices, were connected by horizontal osteotomy cuts[6].

In 1975, Duker conducted research to evaluate the effects of corticotomy on tooth vitality and the marginal periodontium in beagle dogs. He concluded that preserving the marginal bone was essential and that interdental cuts should be made at least 2 mm apical to the alveolar crest level[145]. In 1991, Suya et al[146]. refined the supra-apical horizontal osteotomy incision, concluding that a horizontal corticotomy would aid in the luxation of bone blocks. This technique was further enhanced by Wilcko et al., who integrated alveolar augmentation into the corticotomy-assisted orthodontic technique, patenting it as periodontally accelerated osteogenic orthodontics (PAOO). They employed a combination of demineralized freeze-dried bone allograft (DFDBA)/xenograft or a bioabsorbable alloplastic graft for alveolar augmentation, which covered pre-existing fenestrations and increased bucco-lingual thickness[16].

Periodontally Accelerated Osteogenic Orthodontics (PAOO) is applicable in most instances where traditional fixed orthodontic treatments are utilized. This technique has proven effective in managing Class I malocclusions with moderate to severe crowding, Class II malocclusions that require expansion or extractions, and mild Class III malocclusions. The orthodontic specialist is responsible for formulating the treatment strategy, determining which teeth will function as anchorage points and which sections of the dental arch will be expanded or contracted. From this strategy, a detailed prescription for the areas needing corticotomies is developed. Achieving successful results requires precise collaboration between the surgeon and orthodontist. It is advisable for both professionals to undergo joint training in this method to ensure they possess a unified understanding of the technique[34].

The surgical specialist is tasked with evaluating the patient's aesthetic needs and incorporating these into the surgical treatment plan. For instance, in cases where a patient presents with gingival recession in an area that requires corticotomy, it is possible to perform a subepithelial connective tissue graft alongside the PAOO surgery.

In certain instances, it is necessary to establish anchorage prior to initiating the PAOO procedure. This requirement is particularly prevalent in Class II malocclusions that necessitate retraction. The dental arches may exhibit varying degrees of movement requirements. For instance, there may be mild anterior crowding in the mandibular anterior region, while significant expansion is needed in the maxillary arch. In such a scenario, PAOO may be performed on the maxillary arch, whereas traditional orthodontic therapy is employed to address the mandibular arch. Ideally, both arches should be corrected within a similar timeframe.

Orthodontic bracket placement and arch wire activation are generally conducted one week prior to the surgical component of PAOO. Nevertheless, bracketing may be performed up to one to two weeks post-surgery. In instances where complex mucogingival procedures are integrated with PAOO surgery, the absence of fixed orthodontic appliances may facilitate easier manipulation of the flap and suturing. In all scenarios, the initiation of orthodontic force should not be postponed beyond two weeks following surgery. A delay exceeding this period would not capitalize on the limited duration of the RAP. The orthodontist is afforded a restricted timeframe to achieve accelerated tooth movement, typically spanning four to six months, after which finishing movements proceed at a normal pace. Given this constrained period of rapid movement, the orthodontist must promptly advance arch wire sizes, initially engaging the largest arch wire feasible[34].

PRINCIPLE OF PAOO

It is based on the principle of Regional Acceleratory Phenomena (RAP). Regional Acceleratory Phenomena refers to a localized response to a noxious stimulus, characterized by a process in which tissue formation occurs at a rate surpassing the normal regional regeneration process. By facilitating the various stages of healing, this phenomenon accelerates healing by a factor of 2–10 times compared to normal physiological healing (Frost, 1983)[7]. Numerous studies have documented an increase in the activity of inflammatory markers, such as chemokines and cytokines, in response to orthodontic forces. Chemokines are instrumental in the recruitment of osteoclast precursor cells, while cytokines, either directly or indirectly through the prostaglandin E2 pathway and the RANK/RANKL pathway, facilitate the differentiation of osteoclasts from precursor cells into mature osteoclasts. Consequently, it is reasonable to hypothesize that enhancing the expression of these factors through surgical irritation of the bone could expedite tooth movement[29,147–149].

A histological study demonstrated that selective alveolar decortication induces increased turnover of alveolar spongiosa (Sebaoun et al., 2008). Surgical intervention results in a significant increase in alveolar demineralization, a transient and reversible condition, leading to osteopenia (a temporary decrease in bone mineral density). This osteopenia permits rapid tooth movement, as teeth are supported by and move through trabecular bone. As long as tooth movement persists, RAP is prolonged. Once RAP subsides, osteopenia resolves, and the radiographic appearance of normal spongiosa reemerges. Upon completion of orthodontic tooth movement, an environment conducive to alveolar re-mineralization is established. In essence, surgical irritation of the bone creates a wound that initiates a localized inflammatory response. The presence of inflammatory markers attracts osteoclasts to the area, resulting in bone resorption. This effect, however, is temporary, lasting approximately four months[150], and the procedure may need to be repeated if accelerated tooth movement is still desired.

Technique of periodontally accelerated osteogenic orthodontics

Criteria for Patient Selection[151]

- Class I malocclusion with moderate to severe dental crowding or a constricted maxilla
- Severe bimaxillary protrusion
- Class II malocclusion necessitating maxillary expansion
- Accelerate canine retraction after premolar extraction
- Molar uprighting and intrusion
- Open bite correction
- Facilitation of the eruption of impacted teeth.
- Resolve crowding and shorten treatment time
- Facilitate slow orthodontic expansion
- Manipulation of anchorage
- Enhance post orthodontic stability

Periodontally Accelerated Osteogenic Orthodontics (PAOO) is applicable to both the maxillary and mandibular arches, with the choice of application site guided by clinical judgment. Typically, maxillary expansion demands a longer treatment duration compared to the correction of mild anterior crowding in the mandible. Therefore, in cases where a patient exhibits a narrow maxilla alongside mild anterior crowding, PAOO may be more advantageous in the maxillary arch, while conventional orthodontic methods could be more appropriate for the mandibular arch. Conversely, in scenarios involving bimaxillary dentoalveolar protrusion that necessitates extractions in both arches, PAOO can be utilized to accelerate treatment in both areas. Ideally, achieving simultaneous correction in both arches is preferred for optimal outcomes[151].

Advantages

- Less time than traditional orthodontics
- Less likelihood of root resorption
- History of relapse has been very low
- There is less need for appliances and headgear (depending on the case)
- The technique has its roots in proven orthopedic research and treatments
- Both metal and ceramic brackets can be used

Contraindications

- Patient having active periodontal disease
- Severe class III cases
- Patients having osteoporosis or other bone diseases
- Patients under long-term medication such as NSAIDs
- Patients with systemic diseases

Furthermore, PAOO should not be regarded as a substitute for surgically assisted palatal expansion in the management of severe posterior cross-bite. Additionally, PAOO is not recommended in instances where bimaxillary protrusion is accompanied by a gummy smile, as such cases may derive greater benefit from segmental osteotomy[152].

Surgical stages

The surgical method for Periodontally Accelerated Osteogenic Orthodontics (PAOO) involves five key stages: the elevation of the flap, decortication, the application of particulate grafting, closure, and the subsequent application of orthodontic force.

Flap Design

A well-designed flap is crucial for the success of any surgical procedure. In the context of PAOO, the flap must allow adequate access to the alveolar bone where corticotomies are to be conducted. It is also important to preserve the gingival form to ensure an aesthetically pleasing outcome. The fundamental flap design involves a combination of a full-thickness flap at the most coronal aspect, with a split-thickness dissection in the apical regions[34]. The flap should extend beyond the corticotomy sites mesially and distally, thereby eliminating the need for vertical releasing incisions. For aesthetic considerations, the papilla between the maxillary central incisors should be preserved on both the labial and palatal aspects. Access to the labial alveolar bone in this region is facilitated by "tunneling" from the distal aspect[34]

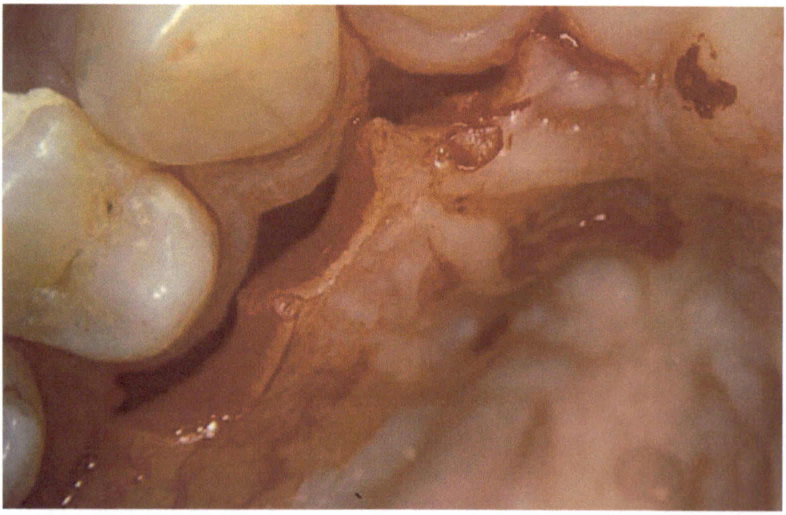

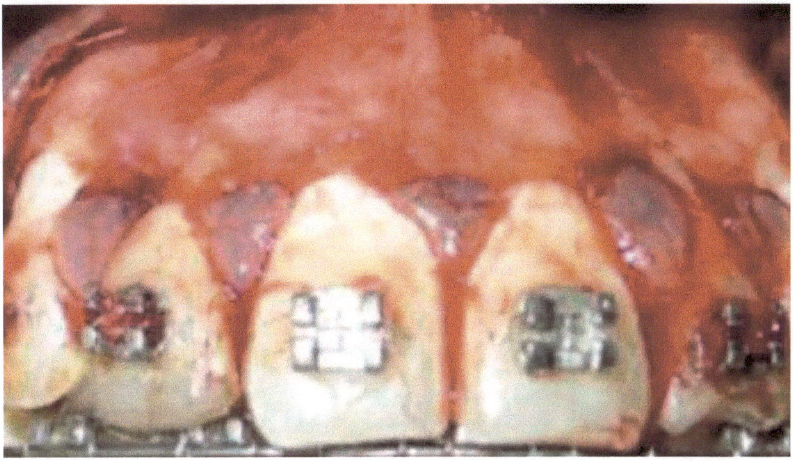

FIG 12: Flap reflection[34,142]

Decortication

Decortication pertains to the excision of the cortical layer of the alveolar bone, ensuring it is adequate to trigger the Regional Acceleratory Phenomenon (RAP) response without resulting in movable bone segments. After the elevation of the flap, decortication of the bone adjacent to malpositioned teeth is performed using low-speed round burs under local anesthesia. In the context of the Periodontally Accelerated Osteogenic Orthodontics (PAOO) procedure, decortication is executed at clinical sites without breaching the cancellous bone, thereby reducing the risk of harm to underlying structures such as the maxillary sinus and the mandibular canal. Corticotomies can also be performed using a piezoelectric knife[153,154]. These corticotomies are strategically placed on both the labial and lingual (palatal) surfaces of the alveolar bone[34].

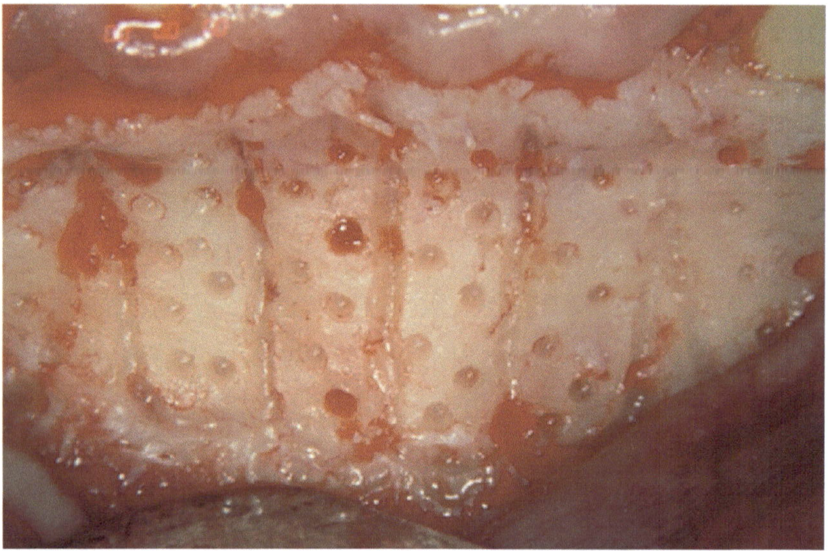

FIG 13: Common decortication scheme[34]

Particulate Grafting

The materials most frequently utilized for grafting following decortication include deproteinized bovine bone, autogenous bone, and decalcified freeze-dried bone allograft, or a combination of these options[34]. Grafting is generally conducted in areas that have undergone corticotomies. The volume of graft material required is influenced by the expected direction and extent of tooth movement, the initial thickness of the alveolar bone, and the necessity for labial support provided by the alveolar bone. Typically, the volume used is between 0.25 and 0.5 ml of graft material per tooth[34].

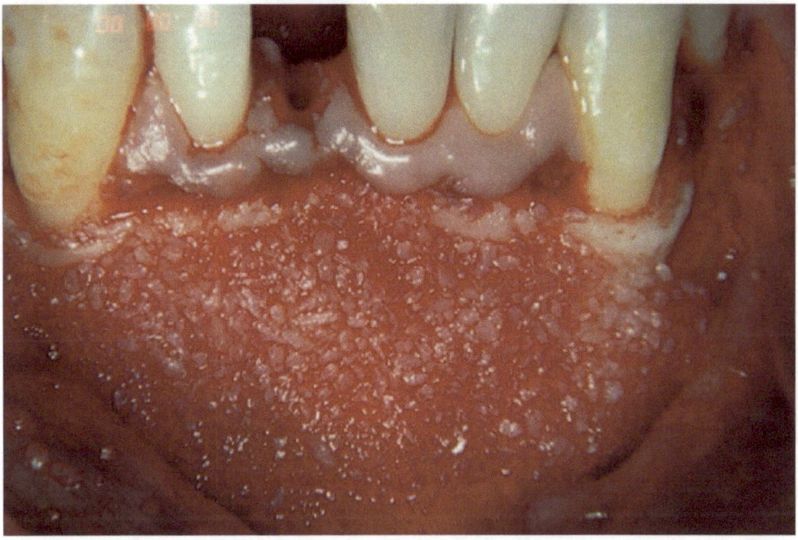

FIG 14: A particulate bone graft was layered over decorticated alveolar bone. The demineralized freeze-dried bone allograft was integrated with activated platelet-rich plasma, producing a gelatinous consistency. This combination improves the handling and physical stability of the graft[34]

Closure Techniques

The flap should be closed using non-resorbable interrupted sutures, ensuring that excessive tension is avoided. Packing is not necessary. The sutures are typically left in place for a duration of 1 to 2 weeks[34].

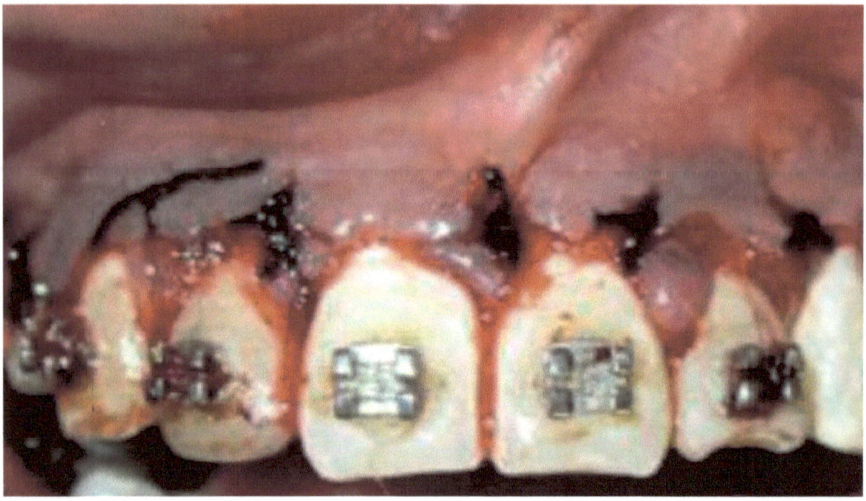

FIG 15: Flap closure[142]

Timing of Orthodontic Treatment

Orthodontic brackets are generally positioned, and arch wires are activated approximately one week before the surgical phase of PAOO. In instances where complex mucogingival procedures are incorporated with PAOO surgery, the absence of fixed orthodontic devices may allow for more straightforward manipulation of the flap and suturing. Once the flap is repositioned, a substantial orthodontic force can be immediately applied to the teeth. It is crucial that the initiation of orthodontic force is not delayed beyond two weeks following surgery, as any delay beyond this period would hinder the optimal utilization of the limited timeframe during which the RAP is active. The orthodontist is tasked with achieving accelerated tooth movement within a constrained period, typically lasting 4 to 6 months, after which the rate of tooth movement returns to normal[34]. To maximize this brief period of rapid movement, the orthodontist should swiftly progress to larger arch wire sizes, starting with the largest feasible arch wire.

Technique Modifications

PAOO can be effectively integrated with gingival augmentation procedures[155]. This approach is particularly crucial for adult patients exhibiting significant gingival recession. In such cases, a subepithelial connective tissue graft is applied over the exposed root surface in conjunction with the placement of particulate graft material. The graft is obtained by excising a 1-2 mm thickness of gingival connective tissue from the elevated palatal flap.

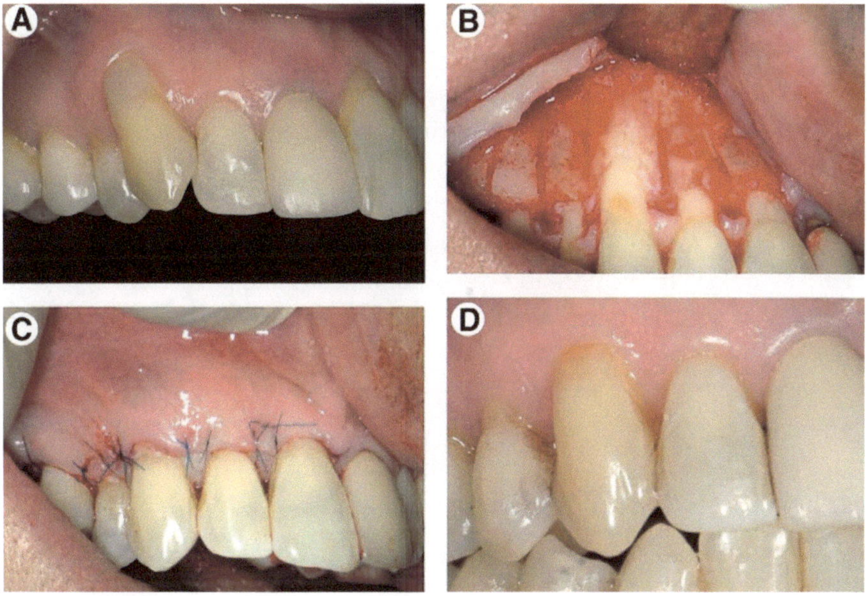

FIG 16: A) Initial assessment of a patient scheduled for a Periodontally Accelerated Osteogenic Orthodontics (PAOO) procedure, exhibiting significant gingival recession on tooth 6. B) Removal of composite restoration followed by the execution of corticotomies. C) Placement of a subepithelial connective tissue graft beneath a coronally advanced flap. D) Outcome observed two years post-surgery[34].

Complications and Adverse effects

While PAOO is generally regarded as a less invasive option compared to osteotomy-assisted orthodontics or surgically assisted rapid expansion, there are documented instances of adverse effects on the periodontium following corticotomy. These effects range from negligible issues to minor interdental bone loss and loss of attached gingiva, with some cases showing periodontal defects, especially when the interdental distance is limited[133,156–158]. Furthermore, subcutaneous hematomas in the facial and neck areas have been reported after intensive corticotomies[10,159]. Post-operative swelling and pain are also anticipated for several days. Notably, there have been no reported negative impacts on the vitality of the dental pulps in the corticotomy region[159].

However, the long-term effects on pulpal vitality after rapid tooth movement have not been thoroughly investigated. An animal study by Liou et al.[160] demonstrated normal pulp vitality following rapid tooth movement at a rate of 1.2 mm per week, indicating the need for further research in this domain.

It is well-established that some root resorption is expected with orthodontic tooth movement[161]. Research has shown a link between increased root resorption and the duration of the applied force[162–164]. The reduced treatment time associated with PAOO may potentially lower the risk of root resorption.

Ren et al.[165] observed rapid tooth movement in beagles post-corticotomy without any root resorption or irreversible pulp injury. Similarly, Moon et al.[166] reported effective maxillary molar intrusion of 3.0 mm in two months using corticotomy combined with a skeletal anchorage system, without root resorption.

MICRO-OSTEOPERFORATIONS

A novel methodology was devised through the examination of the minimal bone trauma necessary to provoke an inflammatory response sufficient to surpass the biological saturation threshold of orthodontic forces, thereby expediting tooth movement without compromising the integrity of the supporting alveolar bone[167].

The proposed technique involves the application of small and shallow osteoperforations, which can be safely executed on the surface of the buccal or lingual cortical plates by the orthodontist, with minimal adverse effects and limited pain or discomfort.

This procedure does not necessitate a soft tissue flap or any additional incisions. In both animal and human studies, the implementation of a few shallow osteoperforations in proximity to the moving tooth resulted in a significant enhancement in inflammation, osteoclast activation, bone remodeling, and tooth movement.

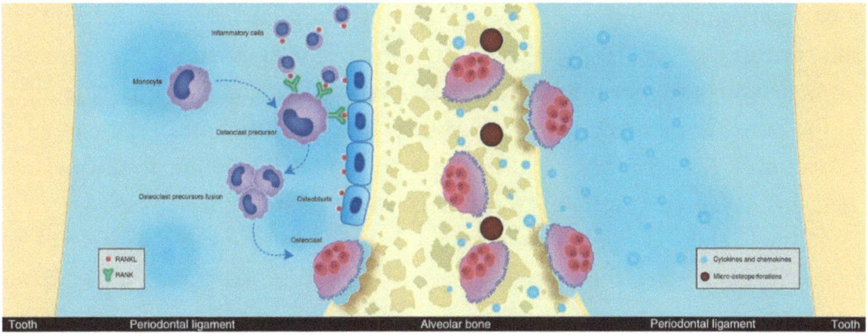

FIG 17: The diagram delineates the roles of cytokines and micro-osteoperforations in the processes of osteoclastogenesis and bone resorption. On the left, it is depicted how inflammatory cells, responding to orthodontic forces, migrate from the bloodstream to the periodontal ligaments. Concurrently, local cells, including osteoblasts, produce nuclear factor κB ligand (RANKL), which interacts with the receptor (RANK) on osteoclast precursor cells such as monocytes. This interaction facilitates the adhesion of these precursor cells, culminating in the formation of osteoclasts that initiate bone resorption. On the right, the application of micro-osteoperforations is shown to amplify the expression of inflammatory cytokines and chemokines, thereby enhancing the recruitment of osteoclasts and subsequently accelerating the bone resorption process[101].

Advantages of Micro-osteoperforations

When evaluating surgical techniques designed to accelerate tooth movement, micro-osteoperforations (MOPs) emerge as a notably advantageous option. This method is characterized by its minimal invasiveness and the absence of flap elevation, allowing orthodontists to perform it safely. In contrast, techniques such as corticotomy or piezoincision require the elevation of a full-thickness flap to reveal the buccal and lingual alveolar bone or necessitate soft tissue incisions followed by interdental cuts through the cortical bone.

A recent adaptation of this approach involves selective decortication in the form of lines and points, with the subsequent application of a resorbable bone graft at the surgical site. The success of this method has been mistakenly linked to the configuration of the bone cuts (block concept) and the bone grafts[16,30,155,168,169]. The progression of tooth movement is primarily influenced by the recruitment and activation of osteoclasts. Thus, regardless of the cut's shape or extent, bone resorption is contingent upon osteoclast activation. This suggests that, similar to micro-osteoperforations, the efficacy of corticotomy or piezoincision is related to the activation of cytokines released due to the trauma induced by the cuts. The cytokine release is expected to be more pronounced in corticotomy and piezoincision compared to micro-osteoperforations, given the more invasive nature and greater trauma to the bone.

However, as with micro-osteoperforations, the elevated cytokine levels are not sustained over a prolonged period and will eventually normalize. Consequently, repeating these procedures to maintain the desired cytokine activity level demands significant financial and time investment from the patient, as it requires the expertise of another specialist, such as a periodontist or oral surgeon.

Alveocentesis

This procedure, termed Alveocentesis, literally translates to puncturing bone.

PROPEL Inc. has engineered a tool designed to enhance the application of MOPs. This instrument enables clinicians to adjust the cutting tip to a specific length, ensuring a safe and predictable procedure based on their clinical evaluation of each patient's periodontal support thickness. The tools are available in both manual and slow-speed handpiece attachments, accommodating situations where dense cortical bone may impede proper penetration. In most cases, straight tools that provide access to the buccal cortical plate with direct vision are adequate. However, for accessing the mandibular lingual plate or the buccal cortical plate near the second molar, a contra-angle tool may be more appropriate.

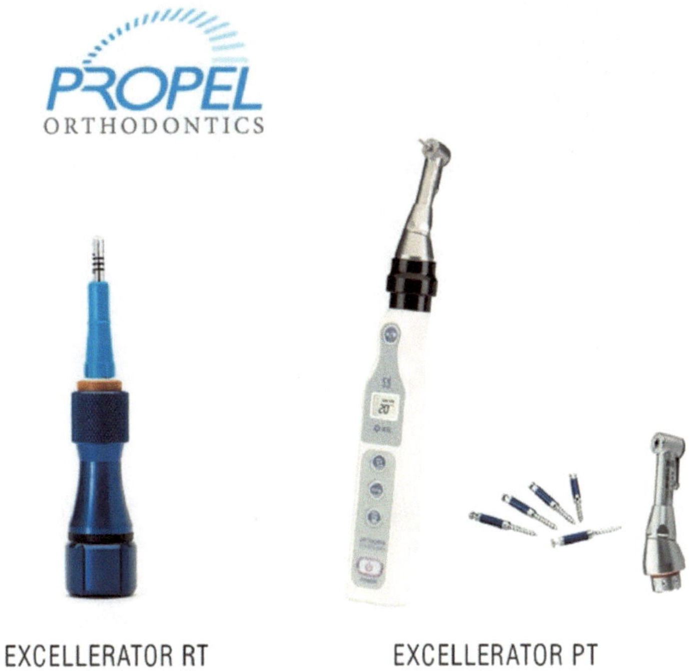

FIG 18: Micro-osteoperforation (MOP) tools, developed by Propel Orthodontics, are available in both manual and rotary formats[101]

This device is a ready-to-use, sterile, disposable instrument. It features an adjustable depth dial and an indicating arrow on the driver body. The adjustable depth dial can be set to 0 mm, 3 mm, 5 mm, and 7 mm of tip depth, contingent upon the area of operation.

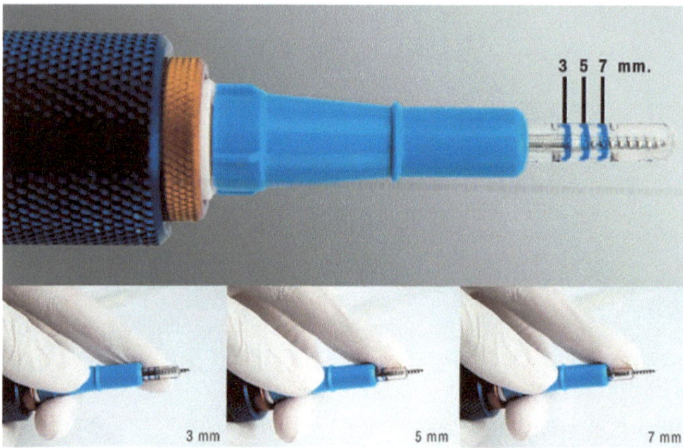

FIG 19: The manual adjustable tool allows setting MOPs length, enabling clinicians to regulate perforation depth according to patient requirements[101]

Previous animal studies have demonstrated that performing micro-osteoperforations (MOPs) on alveolar bone during orthodontic tooth movement can stimulate the expression of inflammatory markers, thereby increase osteoclast activity and accelerate the rate of tooth movement.

In a study conducted by Mani Alikhani et al.[170] in 2013, a single-center, single-blinded design was employed to examine a specific procedure in human subjects. The researchers utilized a Ni-Ti closed coil spring to exert a constant force of 100 g for the distalization of the maxillary canine following the extraction of the first premolar. The spring was anchored to a temporary anchorage device (TAD) positioned distal to the second premolar and connected to the canine via a power arm through the vertical slot of the canine bracket. Gingival crevicular fluid (GCF) samples were collected from each participant to assess the inflammatory response. These samples were obtained prior to orthodontic treatment, immediately before the initiation of canine retraction, and at each subsequent visit between 10 AM and 12 noon.

The samples were collected from the distobuccal crevices of the maxillary canine using filter-paper strips (Oraflow, Smithtown, NY) inserted 1 mm below the gingival margin for 10 seconds. Cytokine levels were quantified using a custom protein array for the following cytokines: CCL 2 (MCP1), CCL-3, CCL-5 (RANTES), IL-8 (CXCL8), IL-1a, IL-1b,

IL-6, and TNF-a (Raybiotech, Norcross, Ga), in accordance with the manufacturer's instructions.

Alginate impressions were obtained at the commencement of the study, immediately prior to canine retraction, and 28 days subsequent to the initiation of canine retraction to monitor the rate of tooth movement. These impressions were promptly cast using plaster (calcium sulfate). Vertical lines were inscribed on the cast over the palatal surface of the canine and lateral incisor, extending from the midpoint of the incisal edge to the midpoint of the cervical line.

The distance between the canine and the lateral incisor was evaluated before and after canine retraction at three specific points: the incisal, middle, and cervical thirds of the crowns. All measurements on the casts were conducted using an electric digital caliper (Orthopli Corp, Philadelphia, Pa) with a precision of 0.01 mm. The study concluded with the assertion that:

1. MOPs significantly enhanced the expression of cytokines and chemokines known to recruit osteoclast precursors and stimulate osteoclast differentiation.
2. MOPs increased the rate of canine retraction by 2.3 times compared to the control group.
3. Patients reported only mild discomfort localized at the site of the MOPs, with minimal to no pain experienced on days 14 and 28.
4. MOPs are deemed an effective, comfortable, and safe procedure to expedite tooth movement during orthodontic treatment.
5. MOPs have the potential to reduce orthodontic treatment duration by 62%.

Catabolic and anabolic bone responses

Micro-osteoperforation is a biologically driven, minimally invasive adjunct in accelerated orthodontics that exerts its effects through a precisely regulated balance between catabolic and anabolic bone responses. The micro-injury produced in the cortical alveolar bone activates the regional acceleratory phenomenon, resulting in a transient but significant increase in bone turnover.

The initial catabolic phase is characterized by an inflammatory response with up-regulation of cytokines and an increased RANKL/OPG ratio, leading to enhanced osteoclast recruitment and activity. This phase produces a localized and reversible osteopenia, effectively reducing the biomechanical resistance of bone to orthodontic forces and thereby facilitating accelerated tooth movement without the need for excessive force application.

Importantly, this resorptive response is not pathological. It is rapidly followed by a biologically coupled anabolic phase, during which osteoblastic activity predominates. Growth factors such as BMPs and TGF-β promote new bone formation, restoration of trabecular architecture, and maturation of bone around the repositioned teeth. This anabolic response ensures maintenance of periodontal integrity, re-establishment of bone density, and long-term stability following tooth movement.

Thus, the clinical success of micro-osteoperforation lies in its ability to harness the body's natural healing mechanisms to create a temporary window of accelerated remodeling, while preserving the equilibrium between bone resorption and formation.

When performed judiciously and combined with optimal orthodontic force systems, MOP provides a safe, predictable, and biologically sound method for reducing treatment time, particularly in adult patients with dense cortical bone.

OBJECTIVES	CLINICAL APPLICATIONS	EFFECT
Accelerating Tooth Movement	Different stages of adult treatment	Catabolic
Facilitating Root Movement / Bodily Movement	Uprighting / Intrusion / Extrusion / Root torque / Closure of large space	Catabolic
Movement into Deficient Alveolar Bone	Closure of old extraction space	Catabolic
Differential Anchorage	Reducing bone density around moving teeth while preserving anchorage unit	Catabolic
Decreased Possibility of Root Resorption	Reducing bone density and duration of exposure to osteoclasts	Catabolic
Restoring Deficient Alveolar Ridge Sinus Remodeling	Tooth movement and cortical drift	Catabolic + Anabolic
Expansion in Adults Asymmetrical Expansion	Cortical drift and bodily movement of buccal segment(s)	Catabolic + Anabolic
Retraction and Protraction Beyond Cortical Boundary	Cortical drift and bodily movement for dental compensation past original plate	Catabolic + Anabolic

LOCATION

Area of Application

The application area of MOPs is contingent upon the clinical indication. To optimize the catabolic effects of MOPs, they should be positioned in proximity to the target teeth while maintaining a distance from the anchor teeth. Consequently, the catabolic effects of MOPs are more localized. For catabolic purposes, deep perforations are typically applied; these perforations are generally executed on the buccal surface between the roots, on the alveolar ridge in cases of extraction, or, less frequently, on the lingual surface between the roots.

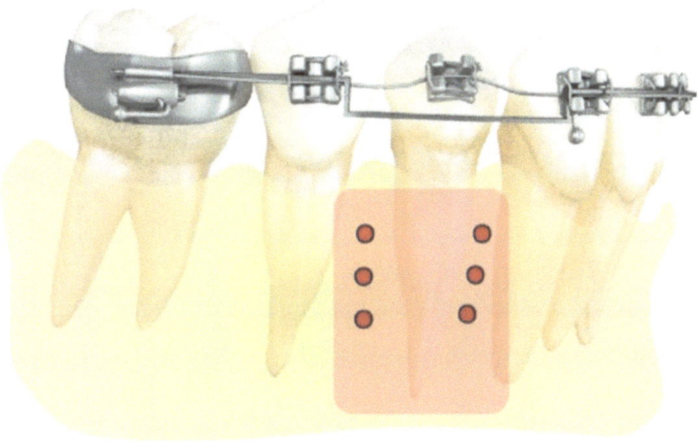

FIG 20: The application of MOPs for catabolic stimulation involves strategically placing perforations mesially and distally to the target tooth within the region of attached gingiva to effectively harness their catabolic effects[101]

To optimize the anabolic effects of MOPs, it is beneficial to increase the coverage of the surface area. As a result, the application area for MOPs to achieve anabolic effects is more widely distributed. To achieve this distribution, shallow perforations can be applied not only between the teeth but also on the bone surface that envelops the roots.

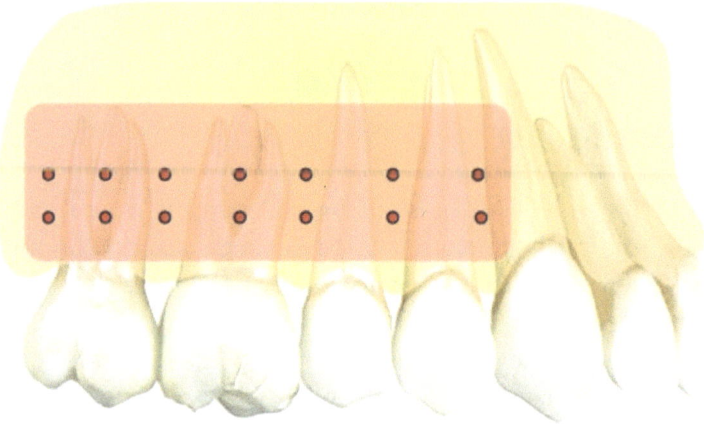

FIG 21: The application of multiple osteoperforations (MOPs) for anabolic stimulation involves the distribution of numerous shallow perforations across the targeted area. This technique is employed to induce an anabolic effect over an extensive periosteal surface[101]

The application area can substantially affect the direction of movement. Within this framework, two clinical scenarios can be identified. In situations where the mechanical design allows for precise force application in a particular direction, the specific placement of MOPs becomes less critical. In these instances, MOPs should be strategically positioned around the target tooth to enhance bone remodeling

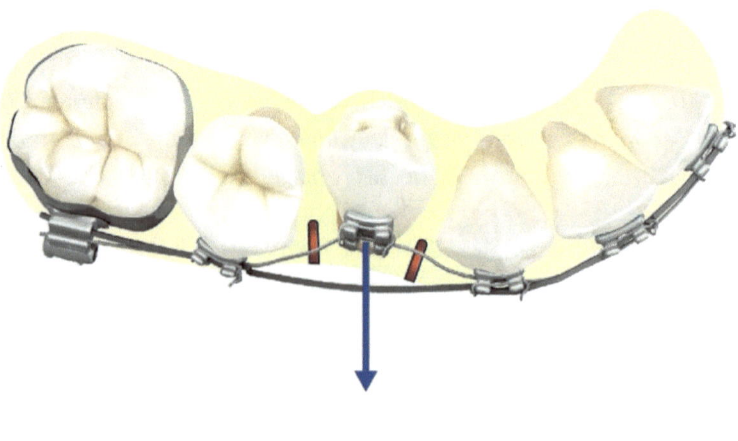

FIG 22: Strategic application of mops based on movement direction. with overlay wire setups, movement direction follows the wire. mops can be applied around the target tooth for buccal movement in direction of blue arrow[101]

Alternatively, directing MOP application in a single direction can effectively promote movement in the desired direction, thereby addressing mechanical limitations in achieving precise movement.

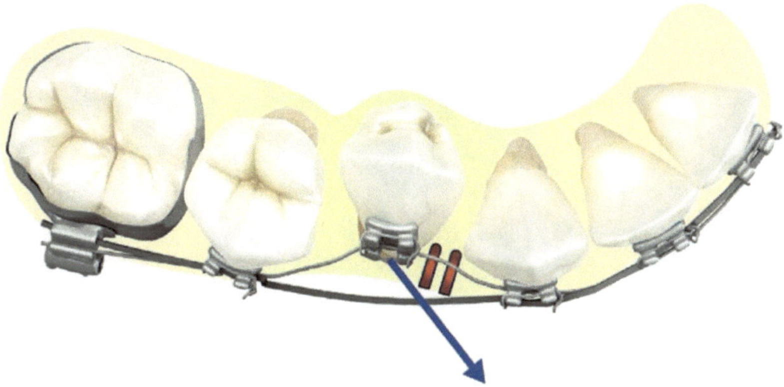

FIG 23: The application of unilateral MOPs facilitates displacement in a specific direction, as indicated by the blue arrow, thereby enabling the clinician to exert greater control over the direction of movement[101]

Height

The optimal placement of MOPs is determined in relation to the mucogingival junction (MGJ). For patient comfort, MOPs should be positioned within the attached gingiva, extending to 1 mm apical to the MGJ. This approach minimizes soft tissue interference during the procedure, reduces postoperative discomfort, and enhances healing. However, in cases where resistance to root movement is encountered, positioning MOPs more apically may be advantageous.

If MOPs are placed in a more apical location, such as for intrusion or torque correction, angling the device apically can be beneficial, allowing access to more apical tissues while still applying MOPs through the attached gingiva. Gripping the bone in this direction is challenging, and the clinician should adjust the appliance if the tool tip slides along the cortical plate. If MOP application through attached gingiva is not feasible, application through mobile mucosa may be considered. Proper lip and cheek retraction to stretch the soft tissues can help prevent ulceration.

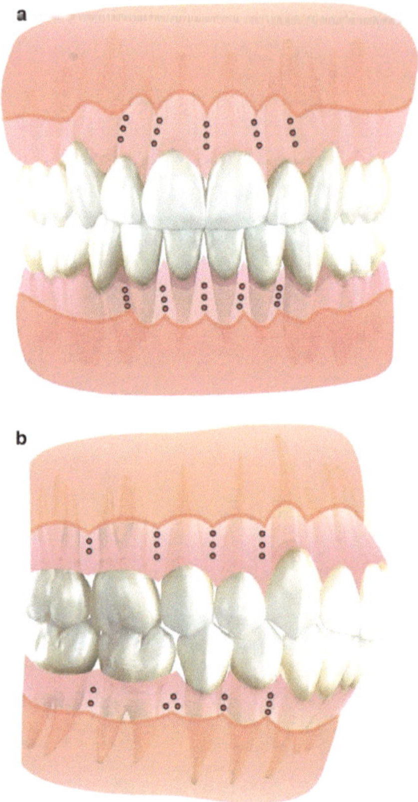

FIG 24: Application of MOPs in the buccal cortical plate. Height of application of MOPs should be limited to attached gingiva for patient comfort. (a) Height of application of MOPs around anterior teeth, (b) application of MOPs around posterior teeth may have different distribution and number as determined by root proximity, accessibility, and width of attached gingiva[101]

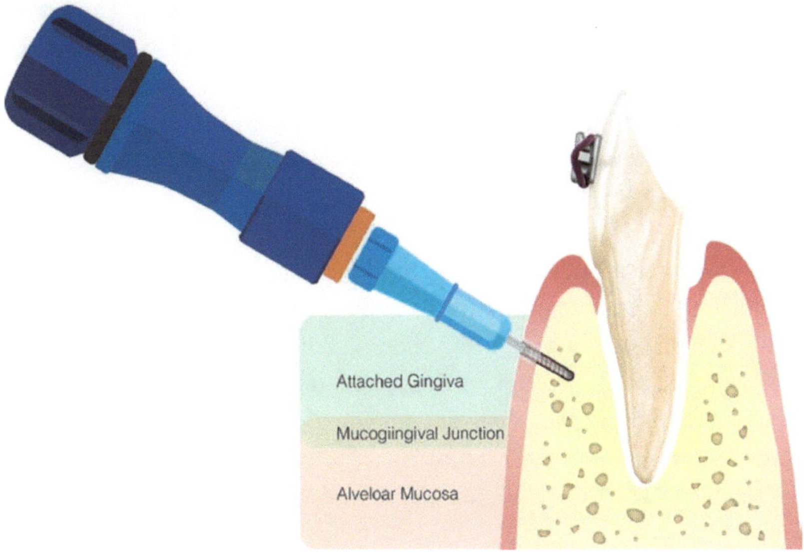

FIG 25: The application of Micro-Osteoperforations (MOPs) can facilitate root movement. When the attached gingiva is narrow, it is feasible to adjust the angle of the MOP device such that the perforation originates from the attached gingiva, while the perforation itself is executed in closer proximity to the root of the tooth[101]

Mesiodistal Position

In the context of deep perforations, which are associated with catabolic effects, the roots delineate the mesiodistal boundaries for the placement of micro-osteoperforations (MOPs). It is imperative to consider the root location and angulation during the execution of MOPs, utilizing the patient's radiographs as a reference. By integrating visualization and palpation of the bone, clinicians can accurately ascertain the root location, thereby identifying the optimal site for MOP placement. Generally, MOPs should be positioned mesially and distally relative to the root of the tooth intended for movement. Instruments designed for MOP application are constructed to avoid root penetration. Should the MOP device's tip approach the roots, the patient will exhibit an immediate response due to hypersensitivity. Furthermore, the device is incapable of further penetration into the root, and a simple retraction and redirection of the device will rectify the issue. In the case of shallow perfortions, which are linked to anabolic effects, MOPs may be applied at any point within the area of interest. Given their purpose of inducing periosteal stimulation, these perforations are superficial, thereby minimizing the likelihood of root contact.

Buccal/Lingual Placement

Micro-osteoperforations (MOPs) can be implemented on both the buccal and lingual cortical plates. However, due to issues related to accessibility, direct visualization, and the thin mucosa covering the lingual cortical plate of the mandible, the buccal cortical plate is generally the preferred site for anterior mandibular MOP placement. Nonetheless, when the lingual cortical plate influences tooth movement or when the anabolic effects of MOPs on the lingual cortical plate are necessary, MOPs should be applied to the lingual plate.

For this application, contra-angle appliances are recommended. In instances of residual ridges, particularly where bone resorption has significantly reduced the width and height of the alveolar bone, MOP application on the ridge's crest is advisable. It is crucial to note that due to bone resorption, vital anatomical structures such as nerves or salivary glands may be more susceptible to trauma; therefore, clinicians should thoroughly examine the area before applying MOPs.

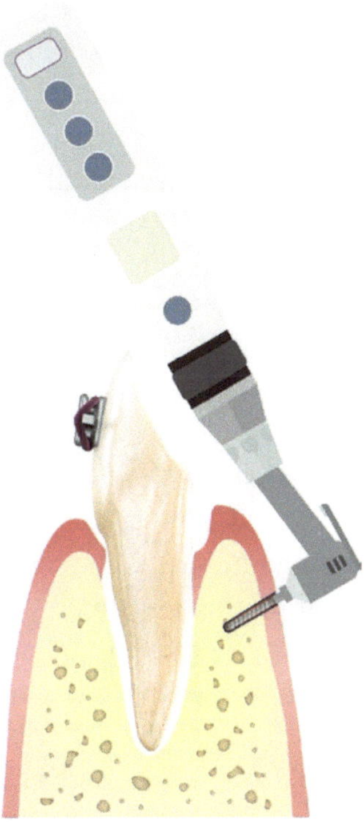

FIG 26: Contra-angle devices, whether manual or rotary, are employed to access the lingual cortical plates and the posterior buccal cortical surfaces. These devices also facilitate the perforation of dense bone that may resist the use of handheld instruments[101]

Number and Depth of MOPs

Micro-osteoperforations (MOPs) enhance the inflammatory response, thereby accelerating bone turnover. Empirical evidence indicates that an increase in trauma severity correlates with an amplified inflammatory response. Consequently, MOPs can elicit more substantial inflammatory reactions through two mechanisms:

1. By augmenting the number of perforations
2. By increasing the depth of penetration.

Research has demonstrated that an increase in the number of MOPs correlates with an accelerated rate of tooth movement. However, due to the constrained space available between dental roots, an optimal range of 2–4 perforations per site is recommended. In scenarios where a higher number of MOPs cannot be applied, increasing the depth of perforation can effectively compensate for the reduced number of perforations.

For catabolic objectives, it is advisable to employ deep micro-osteoperforations (MOPs) with penetration depths ranging from 3 to 7 mm into the bone. However, clinicians must take into account the thickness of the soft tissue and cortical plate when determining the appropriate depth for perforating the cortical plate.

In patients with particularly thick cortical bone, initial MOPs should be shallow to mitigate excessive discomfort. This stimulation initiates the catabolic phase, which reduces bone density. As bone density changes, the depth of perforation can be increased in subsequent applications without causing significant discomfort to the patient.

If the primary aim of treatment is to achieve an anabolic effect through MOPs, deep penetration is unnecessary; shallow MOPs with a perforation depth of 1 to 2 mm are adequate.

In scenarios where both catabolic and anabolic effects of MOPs are desired, a combination of a few deep perforations (to induce catabolic effects) with multiple shallow perforations (to facilitate cortical drifting) will effectively stimulate both processes.

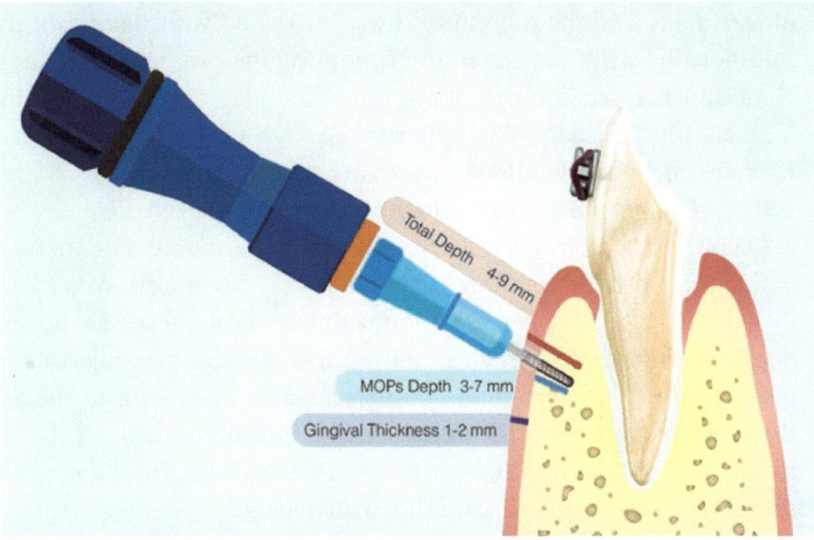

FIG 27: The depth of perforation necessary to achieve a catabolic effect should consider the combined thickness of the soft tissue (1-2 mm) and the bone (3-7 mm) to effectively penetrate the trabecular bone, if feasible. This process may necessitate angling the instrument to circumvent dental roots[101]

Steps in MOPs[101]

1. Instruct the patient to rinse their oral cavity with 15 ml of chlorhexidine oral solution for a duration of 30 seconds.
2. Identify the specific area of interest for the performance of micro-osteoperforations (MOPs). In certain regions, such as the anterior teeth, the utilization of a lip/cheek retractor may facilitate unobstructed access to the MOP application site.
3. Cleanse the area using a damp gauze or cotton roll to remove excess saliva and ensure the area is dry.
4. Administer topical anesthesia to the designated area for anesthetic injection, allowing the topical agent to remain for 1–2 minutes.
5. Initiate local infiltration using a fine needle tip. For MOPs, local infiltration is the sole injection method required for both the maxilla and

mandible. Nerve blocks are unnecessary, as the teeth are not the focus of treatment, and the procedure is not associated with significant pain. Additionally, slight patient awareness during the procedure enables the clinician to ascertain proximity to the roots. The most commonly used local anesthetic is lidocaine (xylocaine) 2% with 1:100,000 epinephrine. In cases of lidocaine allergy, alternatives such as prilocaine 4% with 1:200,000 epinephrine (4% Citanest Forte) or mepivacaine 2% with 1:20,000 levonordefrin (2% Polocaine) may be employed. The anesthetic volume for a single location is approximately one-fourth of a carpule or less. For most procedures, the maximum local anesthesia per visit does not exceed two carpules. Allow a few minutes post-injection and utilize a probe or explorer to verify adequate anesthesia in the area. By anesthetizing only the gingival tissue and periosteum in the area of interest, nociceptive and proprioceptive feedback from the roots is preserved, providing the clinician with biological feedback regarding root or nerve proximity.

6. Prepare a sterile MOP tool equipped with a disposable tip adjusted to the appropriate length. Carefully perforate the cortical plate in the designated area using a gentle, stable rotational motion. Upon reaching the predetermined depth, remove the tool by rotating it in the opposite direction.
7. During the application of MOP, slight bleeding is anticipated. This is a normal occurrence and can be managed by applying pressure to the MOP site with wet gauze or cotton.
8. Prior to discharging the patient, assess the area to ensure that bleeding has ceased. It is recommended that MOPs be administered at the conclusion of the session, allowing the patient to depart subsequently. However, in instances where a fixed orthodontic appliance may impede access, MOPs should be applied following the removal of the wire, after which the patient should be instructed to brush and rinse.

MOP Postoperative Care[101]

Patients who received micro-osteoperforations (MOPs) reported discomfort levels comparable to those experienced by patients who underwent orthodontic force application without MOPs. It is imperative for clinicians to inform patients about the potential for slight discomfort following MOPs. Given the variability in individual responses, patients should be advised to take analgesics, such as acetaminophen, in the event of discomfort. However, the prescription of anti-inflammatory medications, such as nonsteroidal anti-inflammatory drugs (NSAIDs), should be avoided, as these inhibit the inflammatory response essential for the efficacy of MOPs. Postoperative use of chlorhexidine is generally unnecessary; however, it is recommended for patients with poor oral hygiene or compromised health. For most patients, regular mouthwashes or saline rinses suffice to maintain cleanliness in the treated area. There is no need for patients to alter their brushing and flossing habits in the region where MOPs have been applied. Major complications, such as excessive bleeding, infection, or symptomatic root damage, are not anticipated. Nonetheless, clinicians must exercise caution and sound clinical judgment in selecting the location and depth of perforations to prevent unnecessary MOPs. It is crucial to note that MOP tools are single-use and should not be reused, as reuse increases the risk of infection.

CHAPTER VIII

CONCLUSION

Accelerated orthodontics represents a paradigm shift in contemporary orthodontic practice, evolving from purely mechanical tooth movement to a biologically modulated, tissue-responsive approach. The primary objective of accelerated orthodontic techniques is to reduce overall treatment duration while maintaining or enhancing periodontal health, treatment stability, and patient comfort. This is achieved by exploiting the inherent biological capacity of bone and periodontal tissues to remodel rapidly in response to controlled stimuli.

At the core of all accelerated orthodontic modalities lies the concept of enhanced bone turnover, most commonly mediated through the regional acceleratory phenomenon (RAP). Whether induced surgically, mechanically, or biophysically, RAP produces a transient state of localized osteopenia accompanied by increased cellular activity, reduced bone density, and accelerated remodeling. Importantly, this process is reversible and self-limiting, ensuring that rapid tooth movement does not translate into permanent bone loss when techniques are appropriately applied.

Periodontally accelerated orthodontics (PAOO) represents a significant milestone in this evolution by integrating selective alveolar decortication with bone grafting and orthodontic mechanics. PAOO not only accelerates tooth movement through RAP but also expands the envelope of tooth movement by increasing alveolar bone volume. This dual benefit allows for enhanced periodontal support, reduced risk of dehiscence and fenestration, and improved long-term stability. Thus, PAOO exemplifies how acceleration can be achieved without compromising, and in fact enhancing, periodontal health.

Conventional corticotomy-assisted orthodontics further underscores the biological basis of acceleration. By inducing controlled cortical injury, corticotomy stimulates intense osteoclastic activity followed by osteoblastic bone formation, enabling rapid tooth movement. However, its invasive nature has prompted the development of less invasive alternatives that preserve biological efficacy while improving patient acceptance.

In response, minimally invasive techniques such as piezocision and micro-osteoperforation (MOP) have gained prominence. Piezocision utilizes piezoelectric incisions through gingival tissues into cortical bone, selectively triggering RAP while minimizing surgical trauma. Micro-osteoperforation, on the other hand, employs small perforations without flap elevation, inducing localized inflammatory and osteoclastic responses. Both techniques produce a controlled catabolic phase that facilitates tooth movement, followed by an anabolic phase that restores bone integrity. These modalities exemplify the modern trend toward precision-based biological modulation with minimal morbidity.

Parallel to surgical approaches, non-surgical acceleration methods such as low-level laser therapy (LLLT) have expanded the therapeutic spectrum. LLLT accelerates orthodontic tooth movement by enhancing mitochondrial activity, increasing ATP production, and up-regulating cytokines and growth factors that stimulate osteoclastic and osteoblastic activity. Its non-invasive nature, absence of surgical trauma, and favorable patient acceptance make it an attractive adjunct, particularly in patients unwilling or unsuitable for surgical interventions.

Another evolving frontier in accelerated orthodontics is the administration of exogenous biological molecules, including prostaglandins, cytokines, parathyroid hormone, vitamin D metabolites, and growth factors. These agents directly influence cellular signaling pathways involved in bone remodeling, offering the potential for targeted acceleration. While experimental and early clinical results are promising, concerns regarding dosage control, systemic effects, and long-term safety necessitate further research before widespread clinical application.

Collectively, these diverse modalities highlight that accelerated orthodontics is not a single technique but a biologically unified concept employing different methods to achieve the same fundamental goal—enhancement of bone remodeling to facilitate efficient tooth movement. The success of accelerated orthodontics depends not on the magnitude of force applied but on the biological readiness of the supporting tissues to respond to orthodontic forces.

From a clinical standpoint, the judicious selection of acceleration techniques must be individualized based on patient age, periodontal status, systemic health, treatment objectives, and risk–benefit considerations. When properly indicated and executed, accelerated orthodontic procedures do not increase the risk of root resorption, periodontal breakdown, or long-term instability. Instead, they offer the advantages of reduced treatment time, improved patient compliance, and expanded treatment possibilities, particularly in adult orthodontics.

To sum up, accelerated orthodontics represents a harmonious integration of biology, biomechanics, and minimally invasive technology. As understanding of cellular and molecular mechanisms continues to advance, future developments are likely to focus on personalized, targeted, and biologically optimized approaches. Accelerated orthodontics thus stands not merely as a means to shorten treatment duration, but as a refined, evidence-based strategy that enhances the efficiency, predictability, and overall quality of orthodontic care.

Bibliography

1. Nicozisis J. Accelerated orthodontics through micro-osteo- perforation. *Orthodontic Practice US* 2013;4(3):56–7.

2. Tsichlaki A, Chin SY, Pandis N, Fleming PS. How long does treatment with fixed orthodontic appliances last? A systematic review. *Am. J. Orthod. Dentofacial Orthop.* 2016;149(3):308–18.

3. Bhaskar V, Nayak A, Dental T, Orthopaedics D. Accelerated Orthodontics - A Review. 2014. Available at: https://www.semanticscholar.org/paper/Accelerated-Orthodontics-A-Review-Bhaskar-Nayak/51e4876a7741f90be0cdf8c6214017ba7be0b927. Accessed December 8, 2025.

4. Long H, Pyakurel U, Wang Y, Liao L, Zhou Y, Lai W. Interventions for accelerating orthodontic tooth movement: a systematic review: A systematic review. *Angle Orthod.* 2013;83(1):164–71.

5. Li Y, Jacox LA, Little SH, Ko C-C. Orthodontic tooth movement: The biology and clinical implications. *Kaohsiung J. Med. Sci.* 2018;34(4):207–14.

6. Kole H. Surgical operations on the alveolar ridge to correct occlusal abnormalities. *Oral Surg. Oral Med. Oral Pathol.* 1959;12(5):515–29 concl.

7. Frost HM. The regional acceleratory phenomenon: a review. *Henry Ford Hosp. Med. J.* 1983;31(1):3–9.

8. Yamasaki K, Shibata Y, Imai S, Tani Y, Shibasaki Y, Fukuhara T. Clinical application of prostaglandin E1 (PGE1) upon orthodontic tooth movement. *Am. J. Orthod.* 1984;85(6):508–18.

9. Anholm JM, Crites DA, Hoff R, Rathbun WE. Corticotomy-facilitated orthodontics. *CDA J.* 1986;14(12):7–11.

10. Gantes B, Rathbun E, Anholm M. Effects on the periodontium following corticotomy-facilitated orthodontics. Case reports. *J. Periodontol.* 1990;61(4):234–8.

11. Saito M, Saito S, Ngan PW, Shanfeld J, Davidovitch Z. Interleukin 1 beta and prostaglandin E are involved in the response of periodontal cells to mechanical stress in vivo and in vitro. *Am. J. Orthod. Dentofacial Orthop.* 1991;99(3):226–40.

12. Simonet WS, Lacey DL, Dunstan CR, et al. Osteoprotegerin: a novel secreted protein involved in the regulation of bone density. *Cell* 1997;89(2):309–19.

13. Liou EJ, Huang CS. Rapid canine retraction through distraction of the periodontal ligament. *Am. J. Orthod. Dentofacial Orthop.* 1998;114(4):372–82.

14. Collins MK, Sinclair PM. The local use of vitamin D to increase the rate of orthodontic tooth movement. *Am. J. Orthod. Dentofacial Orthop.* 1988;94(4):278–84.

15. Soma S, Matsumoto S, Higuchi Y, et al. Local and chronic application of PTH accelerates tooth movement in rats. *J. Dent. Res.* 2000;79(9):1717–24.

16. Wilcko WM, Wilcko T, Bouquot JE, Ferguson DJ. Rapid orthodontics with alveolar reshaping: two case reports of decrowding. *Int. J. Periodontics Restorative Dent.* 2001;21(1):9–19.

17. Oshiro T, Shiotani A, Shibasaki Y, Sasaki T. Osteoclast induction in periodontal tissue during experimental movement of incisors in osteoprotegerin-deficient mice. *Anat. Rec.* 2002;266(4):218–25.

18. Sekhavat AR, Mousavizadeh K, Pakshir HR, Aslani FS. Effect of misoprostol, a prostaglandin E1 analog, on orthodontic tooth movement in rats. *Am. J. Orthod. Dentofacial Orthop.* 2002;122(5):542–7.

19. Seifi M, Eslami B, Saffar AS. The effect of prostaglandin E2 and calcium gluconate on orthodontic tooth movement and root resorption in rats. *Eur. J. Orthod.* 2003;25(2):199–204.

20. Kale S, Kocadereli I, Atilla P, Aşan E. Comparison of the effects of 1,25 dihydroxycholecalciferol and prostaglandin E2 on orthodontic tooth movement. *Am. J. Orthod. Dentofacial Orthop.* 2004;125(5):607–14.

21. Sayin S, Bengi AO, Gürton AU, Ortakoğlu K. Rapid canine distalization using distraction of the periodontal ligament: a preliminary clinical validation of the original technique. *Angle Orthod.* 2004;74(3):304–15.

22. Cruz DR, Kohara EK, Ribeiro MS, Wetter NU. Effects of low-intensity laser therapy on the orthodontic movement velocity of human teeth: a preliminary study. *Lasers Surg. Med.* 2004;35(2):117–20.

23. Işeri H, Kişnişci R, Bzizi N, Tüz H. Rapid canine retraction and orthodontic treatment with dentoalveolar distraction osteogenesis. *Am. J. Orthod. Dentofacial Orthop.* 2005;127(5):533–41; quiz 625.

24. Nishijima Y, Yamaguchi M, Kojima T, Aihara N, Nakajima R, Kasai K. Levels of RANKL and OPG in gingival crevicular fluid during orthodontic tooth movement and effect of compression force on releases from periodontal ligament cells in vitro. *Orthod. Craniofac. Res.* 2006;9(2):63–70.

25. Goulart CS, Nouer PRA, Mouramartins L, Garbin IU, de Fátima Zanirato Lizarelli R. Photoradiation and orthodontic movement: experimental study with canines. *Photomed. Laser Surg.* 2006;24(2):192–6.

26. Limpanichkul W, Godfrey K, Srisuk N, Rattanayatikul C. Effects of low-level laser therapy on the rate of orthodontic tooth movement. *Orthod. Craniofac. Res.* 2006;9(1):38–43.

27. Kanzaki H, Chiba M, Arai K, et al. Local RANKL gene transfer to the periodontal tissue accelerates orthodontic tooth movement. *Gene Ther.* 2006;13(8):678–85.

28. Krishnan V, Davidovitch Z 'ev. Cellular, molecular, and tissue-level reactions to orthodontic force. *Am. J. Orthod. Dentofacial Orthop.* 2006;129(4): 469.e1–32.

29. Garlet TP, Coelho U, Silva JS, Garlet GP. Cytokine expression pattern in compression and tension sides of the periodontal ligament during orthodontic tooth movement in humans. *Eur. J. Oral Sci.* 2007;115(5):355–62.

30. Fischer TJ. Orthodontic treatment acceleration with corticotomy-assisted exposure of palatally impacted canines. *Angle Orthod.* 2007;77(3):417–20.

31. Youssef M, Ashkar S, Hamade E, Gutknecht N, Lampert F, Mir M. The effect of low-level laser therapy during orthodontic movement: a preliminary study. *Lasers Med. Sci.* 2008;23(1):27–33.

32. Nishimura M, Chiba M, Ohashi T, et al. Periodontal tissue activation by vibration: intermittent stimulation by resonance vibration accelerates experimental tooth movement in rats. *Am. J. Orthod. Dentofacial Orthop.* 2008;133(4):572–83.

33. Kim D-H, Park Y-G, Kang S-G. The effects of electrical current from a micro-electrical device on tooth movement. *Korean J. Orthod.* 2008;38(5):337.

34. Murphy KG, Wilcko MT, Wilcko WM, Ferguson DJ. Periodontal accelerated osteogenic orthodontics: a description of the surgical technique. *J. Oral Maxillofac. Surg.* 2009;67(10):2160–6.

35. Kim S-J, Moon S-U, Kang S-G, Park Y-G. Effects of low-level laser therapy after Corticision on tooth movement and paradental remodeling: LOW-LEVEL LASER THERAPY AND ORTHODONTICS. *Lasers Surg. Med.* 2009;41(7):524–33.

36. Yamaguchi M. RANK/RANKL/OPG during orthodontic tooth movement. *Orthod. Craniofac. Res.* 2009;12(2):113–9.

37. Yamaguchi M, Hayashi M, Fujita S, et al. Low-energy laser irradiation facilitates the velocity of tooth movement and the expressions of matrix metalloproteinase-9, cathepsin K, and alpha(v) beta(3) integrin in rats. *Eur. J. Orthod.* 2010;32(2):131–9.

38. Hassan AH, Al-Fraidi AA, Al-Saeed SH. Corticotomy-assisted orthodontic treatment: review. *Open Dent. J.* 2010;4:159–64.

39. Aboul-Ela SMBE-D, El-Beialy AR, El-Sayed KMF, Selim EMN, El-Mangoury NH, Mostafa YA. Miniscrew implant-supported maxillary canine retraction with and without corticotomy-facilitated orthodontics. *Am. J. Orthod. Dentofacial Orthop.* 2011;139(2):252–9.

40. Kim H-S, Lee Y-J, Park Y-G, et al. Histologic assessment of the biological effects after speedy surgical orthodontics in a beagle animal model: a preliminary study. *Korean J. Orthod.* 2011;41(5):361.

41. Brooks PJ, Heckler AF, Wei K, Gong S-G. M-CSF accelerates orthodontic tooth movement by targeting preosteoclasts in mice. *Angle Orthod.* 2011;81(2):277–83.

42. Baloul SS, Gerstenfeld LC, Morgan EF, Carvalho RS, Van Dyke TE, Kantarci A. Mechanism of action and morphologic changes in the alveolar bone in response to selective alveolar decortication-facilitated tooth movement. *Am. J. Orthod. Dentofacial Orthop.* 2011;139(4 Suppl):S83–101.

43. Kau CH. A radiographic analysis of tooth morphology following the use of a novel cyclical force device in orthodontics. *Head Face Med.* 2011;7(1):14.

44. Doshi-Mehta G, Bhad-Patil WA. Efficacy of low-intensity laser therapy in reducing treatment time and orthodontic pain: a clinical investigation. *Am. J. Orthod. Dentofacial Orthop.* 2012;141(3):289–97.

45. McGorray SP, Dolce C, Kramer S, Stewart D, Wheeler TT. A randomized, placebo-controlled clinical trial on the effects of recombinant human relaxin on tooth movement and short-term stability. *Am. J. Orthod. Dentofacial Orthop.* 2012;141(2):196–203.

46. Shoreibah EA, Salama AE, Attia MS, Abu-Seida SMA-M. Corticotomy-facilitated orthodontics in adults using a further modified technique. *J. Int. Acad. Periodontol.* 2012;14(4):97–104.

47. Kim S-J, Kang Y-G, Park J-H, Kim E-C, Park Y-G. Effects of low-intensity laser therapy on periodontal tissue remodeling during relapse and retention of orthodontically moved teeth. *Lasers Med. Sci.* 2013;28(1):325–33.

48. Nimeri G, Kau CH, Abou-Kheir NS, Corona R. Acceleration of tooth movement during orthodontic treatment--a frontier in orthodontics. *Prog. Orthod.* 2013;14(1):42.

49. Kau CH, Kantarci A, Shaughnessy T, et al. Photobiomodulation accelerates orthodontic alignment in the early phase of treatment. *Prog. Orthod.* 2013;14(1):30.

50. Jofre J, Montenegro J, Arroyo R. Rapid Orthodontics with Flapless Piezoelectric Corticotomies: First Clinical Experiences Ortodoncia Rápida con Corticotomías Piezoeléctricas sin Colgajo: Primeras Experiencias Clínicas. Available at: https://www.scielo.cl/pdf/ijodontos/v7n1/art13.pdf.

51. Keser EI, Dibart S. Sequential piezocision: a novel approach to accelerated orthodontic treatment. *Am. J. Orthod. Dentofacial Orthop.* 2013;144(6):879–89.

52. Genc G, Kocadereli I, Tasar F, Kilinc K, El S, Sarkarati B. Effect of low-level laser therapy (LLLT) on orthodontic tooth movement. *Lasers Med. Sci.* 2013;28(1):41–7.

53. Coscia G, Coscia V, Peluso V, Addabbo F. Augmented corticotomy combined with accelerated orthodontic forces in class III orthognathic patients: morphologic aspects of the mandibular anterior ridge with cone-beam computed tomography. *J. Oral Maxillofac. Surg.* 2013;71(10):1760.e1–9.

54. Ize-Iyamu IN, Saheeb BD, Edetanlen BE. Comparing the 810nm diode laser with conventional surgery in orthodontic soft tissue procedures. *Ghana Med. J.* 2013;47(3):107–11.

55. Kalajzic Z, Peluso EB, Utreja A, et al. Effect of cyclical forces on the periodontal ligament and alveolar bone remodeling during orthodontic tooth movement. *Angle Orthod.* 2014;84(2):297–303.

56. Cao H, Kou X, Yang R, et al. Force-induced Adrb2 in periodontal ligament cells promotes tooth movement. *J. Dent. Res.* 2014;93(11):1163–9.

57. Bhattacharya P, Bhattacharya H, Anjum A, et al. Assessment of corticotomy facilitated tooth movement and changes in alveolar bone thickness - A CT scan study. *J. Clin. Diagn. Res.* 2014;8(10):ZC26–30.

58. Leethanakul C, Kanokkulchai S, Pongpanich S, Leepong N, Charoemratrote C. Interseptal bone reduction on the rate of maxillary canine retraction. *Angle Orthod.* 2014;84(5):839–45.

59. Alikhani M, Alansari S, Sangsuwon C, et al. Micro osteoperforations: Minimally invasive accelerated tooth movement. *Semin. Orthod*

2015;21:162–9.

60. Arakkal JA. Periodontally accelerated osteogenic orthodontics : A surgical technique and case report. *IOSR Journal of Dental and Medical Sciences* 2015;14(12):58–62.

61. Pavlin D, Anthony R, Raj V, Gakunga PT. Cyclic loading (vibration) accelerates tooth movement in orthodontic patients: A double-blind, randomized controlled trial. *Semin. Orthod.* 2015;21(3):187–94.

62. Wu J, Jiang J-H, Xu L, Liang C, Bai Y, Zou W. A pilot clinical study of Class III surgical patients facilitated by improved accelerated osteogenic orthodontic treatments. *Angle Orthod.* 2015;85(4):616–24.

63. Tsai C-Y, Yang T-K, Hsieh H-Y, Yang L-Y. Comparison of the effects of micro-osteoperforation and corticision on the rate of orthodontic tooth movement in rats. *Angle Orthod.* 2016;86(4):558–64.

64. Aksakalli S, Calik B, Kara B, Ezirganli S. Accelerated tooth movement with piezocision and its periodontal-transversal effects in patients with Class II malocclusion. *Angle Orthod.* 2016;86(1):59–65.

65. Leethanakul C, Suamphan S, Jitpukdeebodintra S, Thongudomporn U, Charoemratrote C. Vibratory stimulation increases interleukin-1 beta secretion during orthodontic tooth movement. *Angle Orthod.* 2016;86(1):74–80.

66. Liou EW. The development of submucosal injection of platelet rich plasma for accelerating orthodontic tooth movement and preserving pressure side alveolar bone. *APOS Trends Orthod.* 2016;6(1):5.

67. Park YG. Corticision: A flapless procedure to accelerate tooth movement. *Front. Oral Biol.* 2016;18:109–17.

68. Almpani K, Kantarci A. Surgical methods for the acceleration of the orthodontic tooth movement. *Front. Oral Biol.* 2016;18:92–101.

69. Abbas NH, Sabet NE, Hassan IT. Evaluation of corticotomy-facilitated orthodontics and piezocision in rapid canine retraction. *Am. J. Orthod. Dentofacial Orthop.* 2016;149(4):473–80.

70. Charavet C, Lecloux G, Bruwier A, et al. Localized piezoelectric alveolar decortication for orthodontic treatment in adults: A randomized controlled trial: A randomized controlled trial. *J. Dent. Res.* 2016;95(9):1003–9.

71. Cheung T, Park J, Lee D, et al. Ability of mini-implant-facilitated micro-osteoperforations to accelerate tooth movement in rats. *Am. J. Orthod. Dentofacial Orthop.* 2016;150(6):958–67.

72. Shaughnessy T, Kantarci A, Kau CH, Skrenes D, Skrenes S, Ma D. Intraoral photobiomodulation-induced orthodontic tooth alignment: a preliminary study. *BMC Oral Health* 2016;16(1):3.

73. Munoz F, Jiménez C, Espinoza D, Vervelle A, Beugnet J, Haidar Z. Use of leukocyte and platelet-rich fibrin (L-PRF) in periodontally accelerated osteogenic orthodontics (PAOO): Clinical effects on edema and pain. *J. Clin. Exp. Dent.* 2016;8(2):e119–24.

74. AlSayed Hasan MMA, Sultan K, Hamadah O. Low-level laser therapy effectiveness in accelerating orthodontic tooth movement: A randomized controlled clinical trial. *Angle Orthod.* 2017;87(4):499–504.

75. Alfawal AMH, Hajeer MY, Ajaj MA, Hamadah O, Brad B. Evaluation of piezocision and laser-assisted flapless corticotomy in the acceleration of canine retraction: a randomized controlled trial. *Head Face Med.* 2018;14(1):4.

76. Attri S, Mittal R, Batra P, et al. Comparison of rate of tooth movement and pain perception during accelerated tooth movement associated with conventional fixed appliances with micro-osteoperforations - a randomised controlled trial. *J. Orthod.* 2018;45(4):225–33.

77. Gil APS, Haas OL Jr, Méndez-Manjón I, et al. Alveolar corticotomies for accelerated orthodontics: A systematic review. *J. Craniomaxillofac. Surg.* 2018;46(3):438–45.

78. Varella AM, Revankar AV, Patil AK. Low-level laser therapy increases interleukin-1β in gingival crevicular fluid and enhances the rate of orthodontic tooth movement. *Am. J. Orthod. Dentofacial Orthop.* 2018;154(4):535–44.e5.

79. Sivarajan S, Doss JG, Papageorgiou SN, Cobourne MT, Wey MC. Mini-implant supported canine retraction with micro-osteoperforation: A split-mouth randomized clinical trial. *Angle Orthod.* 2019;89(2):183–9.

80. Aboalnaga AA, Salah Fayed MM, El-Ashmawi NA, Soliman SA. Effect of micro-osteoperforation on the rate of canine retraction: a split-mouth randomized controlled trial. *Prog. Orthod.* 2019;20(1):21.

81. Babanouri N, Ajami S, Salehi P. Effect of mini-screw-facilitated micro-osteoperforation on the rate of orthodontic tooth movement: a single-center, split-mouth, randomized, controlled trial. *Prog. Orthod.* 2020;21(1):7.

82. Narkhede KP, Bhad W, Chavan SJ. Platelet-rich plasma: Its applications in orthodontics – A systematic review. *APOS Trends Orthod.* 2021;11(235):235–46.

83. Bhad Patil WA, Karemore AA. Efficacy of pulsed electromagnetic field in reducing treatment time: A clinical investigation. *Am. J. Orthod. Dentofacial Orthop.* 2022;161(5):652–8.

84. Bilello G, Fazio M, Currò G, Scardina GA, Pizzo G. The effects of low-frequency vibration on aligner treatment duration: A clinical trial: A clinical trial. *J. Int. Soc. Prev. Community Dent.* 2022;12(3):345–52.

85. Güray Y, Yüksel AS. Effect of light-emitting photobiomodulation therapy on the rate of orthodontic tooth movement : A randomized controlled clinical trial. *J. Orofac. Orthop.* 2023;84(Suppl 3):186–99.

86. Shaadouh RI, Hajeer MY, Awawdeh MA, Jaber ST, Mahmoud GA, Almasri I-A. Effectiveness of low-intensity electrical current in accelerating the en-masse retraction of the upper anterior teeth following first-premolar extraction in young adult patients with Class II division 1 malocclusion: A randomized controlled clinical trial. *Int. Orthod.* 2024;22(4):100921.

87. Mousa MM, Hajeer MY, Alam MK, Aljabban O, Almahdi WH. Evaluation of low-level laser therapy and piezocision in the en-masse retraction of upper anterior teeth. *Eur. J. Orthod.* 2025;47(3). Available at: http://dx.doi.org/10.1093/ejo/cjaf026.

88. Burstone CJ, Tanne K. Biomechanical basis of tooth movement. *Nihon Kyosei Shika Gakkai Zasshi* 1986;45(4):541–51.

89. Bartzela T, Türp JC, Motschall E, Maltha JC. Medication effects on the rate of orthodontic tooth movement: a systematic literature review. *Am. J. Orthod. Dentofacial Orthop.* 2009;135(1):16–26.

90. Davidovitch Z, Nicolay OF, Ngan PW, Shanfeld JL. Neurotransmitters, cytokines, and the control of alveolar bone remodeling in orthodontics. *Dent. Clin. North Am.* 1988;32(3):411–35.

91. Kohli SS, Kohli VS. Role of RANKL-RANK/osteoprotegerin molecular complex in bone remodeling and its immunopathologic implications. *Indian J. Endocrinol. Metab.* 2011;15(3):175–81.

92. Udagawa N, Takahashi N, Jimi E, et al. Osteoblasts/stromal cells stimulate osteoclast activation through expression of osteoclast differentiation factor/RANKL but not macrophage colony-stimulating factor: receptor activator of NF-kappa B ligand. *Bone* 1999;25(5):517–23.

93. Kanzaki H, Chiba M, Takahashi I, Haruyama N, Nishimura M, Mitani H. Local OPG gene transfer to periodontal tissue inhibits orthodontic tooth movement. *J. Dent. Res.* 2004;83(12):920–5.

94. Yamasaki K, Miura F, Suda T. Prostaglandin as a mediator of bone resorption induced by experimental tooth movement in rats. *J. Dent. Res.*

1980;59(10):1635–42.

95. Yamasaki K, Shibata Y, Fukuhara T. The effect of prostaglandins on experimental tooth movement in monkeys (Macaca fuscata). *J. Dent. Res.* 1982;61(12):1444–6.

96. Leiker BJ, Nanda RS, Currier GF, Howes RI, Sinha PK. The effects of exogenous prostaglandins on orthodontic tooth movement in rats. *Am. J. Orthod. Dentofacial Orthop.* 1995;108(4):380–8.

97. Takano-Yamamoto T, Kawakami M, Yamashiro T. Effect of age on the rate of tooth movement in combination with local use of 1,25(OH)2D3 and mechanical force in the rat. *J. Dent. Res.* 1992;71(8):1487–92.

98. Suda T, Ueno Y, Fujii K, Shinki T. Vitamin D and bone: Vitamin D and Bone. *J. Cell. Biochem.* 2003;88(2):259–66.

99. Nicozisis JL, Nah-Cederquist H-D, Tuncay OC. Relaxin affects the dentofacial sutural tissues. *Clin. Orthod. Res.* 2000;3(4):192–201.

100. Madan MS, Liu ZJ, Gu GM, King GJ. Effects of human relaxin on orthodontic tooth movement and periodontal ligaments in rats. *Am. J. Orthod. Dentofacial Orthop.* 2007;131(1):8.e1–10.

101. Alikhani M ed. *Clinical guide to accelerated orthodontics: With a focus on micro-osteoperforations.* 1st ed. Cham, Switzerland: Springer International Publishing; 2017.

102. Alikhani M, Alyami B, Lee IS, et al. Saturation of the biological response to orthodontic forces and its effect on the rate of tooth movement. *Orthod. Craniofac. Res.* 2015;18 Suppl 1:8–17.

103. Tweedle JA. The effect of local heat on tooth movement. *Angle Orthod.* 1965;35:218–25.

104. Miyoshi K, Igarashi K, Saeki S, Shinoda H, Mitani H. Tooth movement and changes in periodontal tissue in response to orthodontic force in rats vary depending on the time of day the force is applied. *Eur. J. Orthod.* 2001;23(4):329–38.

105. Beeson DC, Johnston LE, Wisotzky J. Effect of constant currents on orthodontic tooth movement in the cat. *J. Dent. Res.* 1975;54(2):251–4.

106. Davidovitch Z, Finkelson MD, Steigman S, Shanfeld JL, Montgomery PC, Korostoff E. Electric currents, bone remodeling, and orthodontic tooth movement. II. Increase in rate of tooth movement and periodontal cyclic nucleotide levels by combined force and electric current. *Am. J. Orthod.* 1980;77(1):33–47.

107. Blechman AM. Pain-free and mobility-free orthodontics? *Am. J. Orthod. Dentofacial Orthop.* 1998;113(4):379–83.

108. Tengku BS, Joseph BK, Harbrow D, Taverne AA, Symons AL. Effect of a static magnetic field on orthodontic tooth movement in the rat. *Eur. J. Orthod.* 2000;22(5):475–87.

109. Stark TM, Sinclair PM. Effect of pulsed electromagnetic fields on orthodontic tooth movement. *Am. J. Orthod. Dentofacial Orthop.* 1987;91(2):91–104.

110. Dogru M, Akpolat V, Dogru AG, Karadede B, Akkurt A, Karadede MI. Examination of extremely low frequency electromagnetic fields on orthodontic tooth movement in rats. *Biotechnol. Biotechnol. Equip.* 2014;28(1):118–22.

111. Shingade M, Maurya R, Mishra H, Singh H, Agrawal K. Accelerated Orthodontics: A paradigm shift. *Indian J. Orthod. Dentofac. Res.* 2017;3(2):64–8.

112. Camacho AD, Velásquez Cujar SA. Dental movement acceleration: Literature review by an alternative scientific evidence method. *World J. Methodol.* 2014;4(3):151–62.

113. Shaadouh RI, Hajeer MY, Al-Sabbagh R, Alam MK, Mahmoud G, Idris G. A novel method to accelerate orthodontic tooth movement using low-intensity direct electrical current in patients requiring en-Masse retraction of the upper anterior teeth: A preliminary clinical report. *Cureus* 2023;15(5):e39438.

114. Huang Y-Y, Chen AC-H, Carroll JD, Hamblin MR. Biphasic dose response in low level light therapy. *Dose Response* 2009;7(4):358–83.

115. Bjordal JM, Lopes-Martins RA, Joensen J, et al. A systematic review with procedural assessments and meta-analysis of low level laser therapy in lateral elbow tendinopathy (tennis elbow). *BMC Musculoskelet. Disord.* 2008;9(1):75.

116. Bjordal JM, Couppé C, Chow RT, Tunér J, Ljunggren EA. A systematic review of low level laser therapy with location-specific doses for pain from chronic joint disorders. *Aust. J. Physiother.* 2003;49(2):107–16.

117. Chow RT, Johnson MI, Lopes-Martins RAB, Bjordal JM. Efficacy of low-level laser therapy in the management of neck pain: a systematic review and meta-analysis of randomised placebo or active-treatment controlled trials. *Lancet* 2009;374(9705):1897–908.

118. Kawasaki K, Shimizu N. Effects of low-energy laser irradiation on bone remodeling during experimental tooth movement in rats. *Lasers Surg. Med.* 2000;26(3):282–91.

119. Marquezan M, Bolognese AM, Araújo MT de S. Effects of two low-intensity laser therapy protocols on experimental tooth movement. *Photomed. Laser Surg.* 2010;28(6):757–62.

120. Fujita S, Yamaguchi M, Utsunomiya T, Yamamoto H, Kasai K. Low-energy laser stimulates tooth movement velocity via expression of RANK and RANKL. *Orthod. Craniofac. Res.* 2008;11(3):143–55.

121. Patil K, Singh Maan A, Orthodontics A. *Current Approaches in Orthodontics IntechOpen.*; 2019.

122. Bjordal JM, Johnson MI, Iversen V, Aimbire F, Lopes-Martins RAB. Low-level laser therapy in acute pain: a systematic review of possible mechanisms of action and clinical effects in randomized placebo-controlled trials. *Photomed. Laser Surg.* 2006;24(2):158–68.

123. Na S, TruongVo T, Jiang F, et al. Dose analysis of photobiomodulation therapy on osteoblast, osteoclast, and osteocyte. *J. Biomed. Opt.* 2018;23(7):1–8.

124. Cotomacio CC, Calarga CC, Yshikawa BK, Arana-Chavez VE, Simões A. Wound healing process with different photobiomodulation therapy protocols to treat 5-FU-induced oral mucositis in hamsters. *Arch. Oral Biol.* 2021;131(105250):105250.

125. Meikle MC. The tissue, cellular, and molecular regulation of orthodontic tooth movement: 100 years after Carl Sandstedt. *Eur. J. Orthod.* 2006;28(3):221–40.

126. K. Patil A, Singh Maan A. Accelerated Orthodontics. In: *Current Approaches in Orthodontics* IntechOpen; 2019.

127. Proffit WR, Fields HW, Sarver DM. *Contemporary Orthodontics Online.* 4th ed. St. Louis, MO: Mosby; 2006. Available at: https://books.google.com/books?id=A45nDwAAQBAJ&newbks=1.

128. Erverdi N, Küçükkeleş N, Şener C, Selamet BU. Interdental distraction osteogenesis for the management of alveolar clefts: archwise distraction. *Int. J. Oral Maxillofac. Surg.* 2012;41(1):37–41.

129. Sukurica Y, Karaman A, Gürel HG, Dolanmaz D. Rapid canine distalization through segmental alveolar distraction osteogenesis. *Angle Orthod.* 2007;77(2):226–36.

130. Lee W. Corticotomy for orthodontic tooth movement. *J. Korean Assoc. Oral Maxillofac. Surg.* 2018;44(6):251–8.

131. Alghamdi AST. Corticotomy facilitated orthodontics: Review of a technique. *Saudi Dent. J.* 2010;22(1):1–5.

132. Buschang PH, Campbell PM, Ruso S. Accelerating tooth movement with corticotomies: Is it possible and desirable? *Semin. Orthod.* 2012;18(4):286–94.

133. Wilcko MT, Wilcko WM, Pulver JJ, Bissada NF, Bouquot JE. Accelerated osteogenic orthodontics technique: a 1-stage surgically facilitated rapid orthodontic technique with alveolar augmentation. *J. Oral Maxillofac. Surg.* 2009;67(10):2149–59.

134. Wang L, Lee W, Lei D-L, Liu Y-P, Yamashita D-D, Yen SL-K. Tisssue responses in corticotomy- and osteotomy-assisted tooth movements in rats: histology and immunostaining. *Am. J. Orthod. Dentofacial Orthop.* 2009;136(6):770.e1–11; discussion 770–1.

135. Wilcko MT, Wilcko WM, Bissada NF. An evidence-based analysis of periodontally accelerated orthodontic and osteogenic techniques: A synthesis of scientific perspectives. *Semin. Orthod.* 2008;14(4):305–16.

136. Charavet C, Lambert F, Lecloux G, Le Gall M. Traitement orthodontique accéléré par corticotomies : quelles sont les alternatives minimalement invasives ? *Orthod. Fr.* 2019;90(1):5–12.

137. Qamruddin I, Alam MK, Khamis MF, Husein A. Minimally invasive techniques to accelerate the orthodontic tooth movement: A systematic review of animal studies. *Biomed Res. Int.* 2015;2015:608530.

138. Shenava S, Us Krishna Nayak V. Accelerated Orthodontics - A Review. *International Journal of Scientifi c Study* 2014;1(5):35–9.

139. Dibart S, Yee C, Surmenian J, et al. Tissue response during Piezocision-assisted tooth movement: a histological study in rats. *Eur. J. Orthod.* 2014;36(4):457–64.

140. Fu T, Liu S, Zhao H, Cao M, Zhang R. Effectiveness and safety of minimally invasive orthodontic tooth movement acceleration: A systematic review and meta-analysis. *J. Dent. Res.* 2019;98(13):1469–79.

141. Jofre J, Montenegro J, Arroyo R. *Rapid Orthodontics with Flapless Piezoelectric Corticotomies: First Clinical Experiences Ortodoncia Rápida Con Corticotomías Piezoeléctricas Sin Colgajo.* Primeras Experiencias Clínicas

142. Srivastava A, Gupta S, Singh R, Chourasia S, Sharma P, Singh GB. Wilckodontics: The periodontal orthodontics. *Dent. J. Adv. Stud.* 2019;6(2--3):53–6.

143. K S, M S, D R, Gowd P. Wilckodontics - a novel synergy in time to save time. *J. Clin. Diagn. Res.* 2014;8(1):322–5.

144. Guilford SH. *Orthodontia, or, malposition of the human teeth.* Trieste Publishing; 2018.

145. Düker J. Experimental animal research into segmental alveolar movement after corticotomy. *J. Maxillofac. Surg.* 1975;3(2):81–4.

146. Suya H. *Mechanical and Biological Basis in Orthodontics Therapy.* (Hösl E, Baldauf A, eds.). Heidelberg, Germany: HütligBuch; 1991:107–226.

147. Taddei SR de A, Andrade I Jr, Queiroz-Junior CM, et al. Role of CCR2 in orthodontic tooth movement. *Am. J. Orthod. Dentofacial Orthop.* 2012;141(2):153–60.

148. Uematsu S, Mogi M, Deguchi T. Interleukin (IL)-1 beta, IL-6, tumor necrosis factor-alpha, epidermal growth factor, and beta 2-microglobulin levels are elevated in gingival crevicular fluid during human orthodontic tooth movement. *J. Dent. Res.* 1996;75(1):562–7.

149. Bletsa A, Berggreen E, Brudvik P. Interleukin-1alpha and tumor necrosis factor-alpha expression during the early phases of orthodontic tooth movement in rats. *Eur. J. Oral Sci.* 2006;114(5):423–9.

150. Mathews DP, Kokich VG. Accelerating tooth movement: the case against corticotomy-induced orthodontics. *Am. J. Orthod. Dentofacial Orthop.* 2013;144(1):5–13.

151. Amit G, Jps K, Pankaj B, Suchinder S, Parul B. Periodontally accelerated osteogenic orthodontics (PAOO) - a review. *J. Clin. Exp. Dent.* 2012;4(5):e292–6.

152. Lee J-K, Chung K-R, Baek S-H. Treatment outcomes of orthodontic treatment, corticotomy-assisted orthodontic treatment, and anterior segmental osteotomy for bimaxillary dentoalveolar protrusion. *Plast. Reconstr. Surg.* 2007;120(4):1027–36.

153. Dibart S, Sebaoun JD, Surmenian J. Piezocision: a minimally invasive, periodontally accelerated orthodontic tooth movement procedure. *Compend. Contin. Educ. Dent.* 2009;30(6):342–4, 346, 348–50.

154. Kim S-H, Kim I, Jeong D-M, Chung K-R, Zadeh H. Corticotomy-assisted decompensation for augmentation of the mandibular anterior ridge. *Am. J. Orthod. Dentofacial Orthop.* 2011;140(5):720–31.

155. Wilcko MT, Wilcko WM, Murphy KG, et al. Full-thickness flap/subepithelial connective tissue grafting with intramarrow penetrations: three case reports of lingual root coverage. *Int. J. Periodontics Restorative Dent.* 2005;25(6):561–9.

156. Iino S, Sakoda S, Miyawaki S. An adult bimaxillary protrusion treated with corticotomy-facilitated orthodontics and titanium miniplates. *Angle Orthod.* 2006;76(6):1074–82.

157. Kwon HJ, Pihlstrom B, Waite DE. Effects on the periodontium of vertical bone cutting for segmental osteotomy. *J. Oral Maxillofac. Surg.* 1985;43(12):952–5.

158. Dorfman HS, Turvey TA. Alterations in osseous crestal height following interdental osteotomies. *Oral Surg. Oral Med. Oral Pathol.* 1979;48(2):120–5.

159. Oztürk M, Doruk C, Ozeç I, Polat S, Babacan H, Biçakci AA. Pulpal blood flow: effects of corticotomy and midline osteotomy in surgically assisted rapid palatal expansion. *J. Craniomaxillofac. Surg.* 2003;31(2):97–100.

160. Liou EJ, Figueroa AA, Polley JW. Rapid orthodontic tooth movement into newly distracted bone after mandibular distraction osteogenesis in a canine model. *Am. J. Orthod. Dentofacial Orthop.* 2000;117(4):391–8.

161. Owman-Moll P, Kurol J, Lundgren D. Continuous versus interrupted continuous orthodontic force related to early tooth movement and root resorption. *Angle Orthod.* 1995;65(6):395–401; discussion 401–2.

162. Harry MR, Sims MR. Root resorption in bicuspid intrusion. A scanning electron microscope study. *Angle Orthod.* 1982;52(3):235–58.

163. Kvam E. Scanning electron microscopy of tissue changes on the pressure surface of human premolars following tooth movement. *Scand. J. Dent. Res.* 1972;80(5):357–68.

164. McFadden WM, Engstrom C, Engstrom H, Anholm JM. A study of the relationship between incisor intrusion and root shortening. *Am. J. Orthod. Dentofacial Orthop.* 1989;96(5):390–6.

165. Ren A, Lv T, Kang N, Zhao B, Chen Y, Bai D. Rapid orthodontic tooth movement aided by alveolar surgery in beagles. *Am. J. Orthod. Dentofacial Orthop.* 2007;131(2):160.e1–10.

166. Moon C-H, Wee J-U, Lee H-S. Intrusion of overerupted molars by corticotomy and orthodontic skeletal anchorage. *Angle Orthod.* 2007;77(6):1119–25.

167. Teixeira CC, Khoo E, Tran J, et al. Cytokine expression and accelerated tooth movement. *J. Dent. Res.* 2010;89(10):1135–41.

168. Wilcko MT, Wilcko WM, Pulver JJ, Bissada NF, Bouquot JE. Accelerated osteogenic ortho dontics technique: a 1-stage surgically facilitated rapid orthodontic technique with alveolar augmentation. *J Oral Maxillofac Surg* 2009;67(10):2149–59.

169. Nowzari H, Yorita FK, Chang H-C. Periodontally accelerated osteogenic orthodontics combined with autogenous bone grafting. *Compend. Contin. Educ. Dent.* 2008;29(4):200–6; quiz 207, 218.

170. Alikhani M, Raptis M, Zoldan B, et al. Effect of micro-osteoperforations on the rate of tooth movement. *Am. J. Orthod. Dentofacial Orthop.* 2013;144(5):639–48.

www.ingramcontent.com/pod-product-compliance
Lightning Source LLC
LaVergne TN
LVHW051129210926
848482LV00001B/25
* 9 7 9 8 9 0 5 1 0 0 4 2 0 *